Senior Encores

William N. Hosley, Sr.

Senior Encores

A Guide to Fulfillment in the Third Age of Life

toExcel

San Jose New York Lincoln Shanghai

Senior Encores

A Guide to Fulfillment in the Third Age of Life

Published by toExcel,
an imprint of iUniverse.com, Inc.

For information address:
iUniverse.com, Inc.
620 North 48th Street
Suite 201
Lincoln, NE 68504-3467
www.iUniverse.com

ISBN: 1-58348-289-X

LCCN: 99-62739

Printed in the United States of America

PREFACE

This work is the result of a compilation of material for a senior issues forum conducted for community groups in Rochester, New York. The material has been collected from a variety of sources and is presented in response to a desire by persons in the "Third Age" of life to expand their horizons and enhance meaningfulness in their lives. Spirituality has been added to the equation and it is defined broadly and non-religiously. The book explores the relationship of one's spirituality to most aspects of senior life and how it can influence the decisions one makes regarding all sorts of intellectual, economic and physical activities as well as pursuit of opportunities and options. The thoughts expressed are intended to be applicable to persons of all religious faiths and beliefs.

This writing is directed to a cross-section of seniors, ages roughly 60 to 90 both male and female, single or married. It considers that some readers may be fairly fit physically while others may have some disabilities. The book presumes that readers are still reasonably sound mentally and have enough financial resources to accommodate at least a few options for discretionary expenditure.

Most of the material in this work has been derived from the writings, lectures and comments of others. There is little that is new in the issues themselves; seniors have been facing most of them for generations. However, many options and approaches are new, like medical care, activity alternatives and the use of the Internet and e-mail. At age 73, 1 am personally in the midst of many of the concerns expressed in the book. I have tried to bring a focus to all major ideas regarding senior issues and the options available and perhaps add a new perspective to the subject to help make life more fulfilling in today's environment.

I recognize that there may be disagreement with the positions taken in regard to some of the issues. In fact, in a number of instances, a somewhat extreme view has been offered so as to sharpen the issues and suggest debate. It is hoped that such controversy is useful and that there may be lively discussions among readers. The content of the book can serve as a take-off point for church and community discussion groups.

I want to thank the many writers on these subjects from whom I have drawn ideas, especially Herbert Benson, MD; Rabbi Z. Schlacter-Shalomi; psychologist, C. Marrett Lacey, PhD and M. Scott Peck, MD.

Finally and uppermost, I would like to think that the contents of this book might inspire and guide all senior readers to a more fulfilling and meaningful "Third Age" of life.

Wm. N. Hosley, Sr
Rochester, New York
September, 1999

CONTENTS

Relationships with Spouse and Others; Self-Empowerment. Understanding: Mind/Body Interactions and the three-legged Stool of Health Care—Medication, Treatment, Self-help. Information regarding: Nutrition, Diet and Weight Control; Longer and Better Life through Exercise and Physical Activity; Sexual Fulfillment for Seniors.

Planning a Funeral and Disposition of Remains; making a Will and Bequests; Writing an Obituary; executing Living Wills and Health-Care Proxies. For survivors—Dealing with Grief and Finding a New Life.

I

THE THIRD AGE

Since people are Living Longer, as much as 35 years after "retirement", this is the Magnificent Opportunity to redefine oneself. Some suggestions to Avoid the Major Diseases of seniors and improve Longevity.

Social Security was first implemented in 1936 and, when one retired at age 65, life expectancy was about three more years. Antibiotics had not been discovered and pneumonia and infections claimed the lives of many. Even if a person lived longer than age 70, it was often not a comfortable life. Typically, the old folks were dependent upon their children. Frequently they were feeble or troubled by failing hearts, eyes, limbs, minds, hearing, lungs and/or poor circulation. Cancer meant a certain, painful end in the near future. For the vast majority of older persons, the idea of a meaningful "third age" was an unknown and irrelevant concept.

Much has changed. Not only has life expectancy increased greatly in recent decades, but the quality of life for many has improved, thanks to advances in not only medicines and treatment but also to better nutrition and environmental and economic conditions.

The expression, "Third Age", is derived from the concept that life can be viewed as being composed of three stages. The "First Age", roughly from birth to about 30 years old is a time of growing, learning and preparation for the "Second Age", roughly ages 30 to 60, which is thought to be the time for building resources and producing children, goods, services and other good works. The "Third Age" is defined as a time for fulfillment and enjoyment of the resources created in the "Second Age". No one's life is that stereotyped, but the concept helps life-phase definition and recognition.

An alternative expression for Third Age is, of course, one's retirement age. To some, the word, retirement, implies withdrawal and that does not describe those who want to do more with their lives. Many are in good health and have discretionary money and wish to take advantage of the many options available. In the U.S., millions of retired seniors are living active and productive lives making significant contributions to the world. For many, retirement means doing or discovering what they always wanted to do—an epiphany, so to speak.

> The Third Age Media, Inc. of San Francisco suggests that: "The Third Age is the new extended period of active adulthood. It is characterized by a sense of accomplishment and fresh beginnings for individuals who champion a new view of what it means to be older".

> "In my first age", the typical Third Ager says, "I developed into a person. In my second age, I pursued my career and raised my family. Now, in the Third Age of life, I have come into my own. This is my time for creativity, continued learning and explorations. I have energy, resources and a fully developed sense of what I want to do with them. It is my time to enjoy new relationships, appreciate family and friends and explore the spiritual side of life. It is also my time, if I choose, for giving back to society and for sharing the wisdom of my experience.

Third Agers are older adults. They drive and define the Third Age experience for themselves, their peers and individuals entering this phase of life. Third Agers are perfectly capable of navigating their way independently through the age, but may prefer to undertake this journey in the company of their peers.

Words that describe Third Agers include:

self-reliant	experienced	involved
aware of their world	experience seeking	socially aware
savvy	curious	learning
teaching	sharing	self-empowering

Rabbi Zalman Schacter-Shalomi, founder of the Spiritual Eldering Institute has this to say:

> For our generation, aging is a new territory. The tribal and traditional ways which supported our ancestors do not always fit for those of us who work and live in this modern time.

> As I was getting close to my 60th birthday, I began to feel the need to see the panorama of my life. I noticed the pressure of growing older and the depression I felt. What would I do with all the extra years of life?

> It looked to me that I would get to live longer than my grandparents and even longer than my parents. Would the extended lifespan be a blessing or a curse, a drawn out medically dying? What does one do with the extra years?

> As I engaged in a review of my life, I began to feel lighter. I began to see myself becoming an elder. The process of spiritual eldering leads one to become a keeper of wisdom.

> An elder is a sounding board, a father confessor who can listen and mentor and perpetuate the wisdom.

Longevity

Today, in the U.S.A., at age 60, life expectancy is 24 years (plus 2 for women, less 2 for men). At 70, the expectation is 16 more years (plus 1 for women, less 1 for men). If one makes it to age 80, the expectation is for 10 more years and, at 90, it's 5 more, and the expectations are increasing!

These numbers are, of course, the means or central tendency of probability distributions. That is to say that for a group of 60-year olds, half will live beyond age 84 and the other half won't make it that far. In fact, about 15% of 60-year-olds will be gone within about 8 years while another 15% will still be around at age 90. A few will make it to 100 and those numbers are growing every year.

Can the odds be beaten? Is it all a matter of chance? The answer is yes and no. Although it is true that genes are an important organic influence on longevity, there are many factors that a person can control to improve the chances for a longer and more fulfilling Third Age. While we all realize that the Third Age is terminal, we don't want it to end prematurely. Our major premature killers are heart disease, lung cancer, diabetes, colon-rectal cancer, prostate cancer (in men) and breast cancer (in women). If one can avoid or successfully treat these diseases, the chances of beating the longevity averages are improved. The good news is that there are many things that one can do to try to avoid these killers. We will explore them in some detail in later chapters.

It is not enough to live longer. One wants also to live well. To have a fulfilling Third Age, one not only has to be alive to enjoy it, but one must also be fairly healthy, or at least able to cope with disabilities, and be reasonably financially secure. It is the object of this book to help people achieve improved quality of life through suggestions regarding health, finance and spiritual enhancement.

One's longevity chances are often improved by having parents and grandparents who had long lives. If all 4 grandparents lived into their 80's, one's chances of duplicating or exceeding that age are very good. However, most people are descended from a mixture of final ages. Furthermore, the grandparents of today's Third Agers often died young from causes like pneumonia that are now quite treatable thus obscuring how long the grandparents might have lived in today's environment of health care. These unknowns are encouraging though, in that they make it seem that we all have a good chance of improved longevity if we do the "right things". A large part of this book is devoted to a discussion of the "right things".

At the top of the list of right things to do are no smoking, modest alcohol consumption, keeping weight near an ideal level through proper diet and nutrition, regular exercise and proper medical care.

Heart disease and strokes account for about 500,000 premature deaths per year in the United States. Factors that increase one's risk of heart disease are: high blood pressure, high LDL cholesterol, low HDL cholesterol, diets high in fat and cholesterol, sedentary or stressful life style, being significantly overweight (especially in the abdominal area), family history, diabetes and, of course, smoking. If you have a father or brother who had a heart attack before age 55 or a mother or sister that had an attack before age 65, you may have an increased risk. Everyone, especially those at risk for heart disease, should discuss the matter with his or her doctor. If appropriate, the doctor is likely to prescribe cholesterol lowering and/or blood pressure reducing medications. For many people, the doctor may suggest an aspirin every day or two to reduce the danger of blood clot formation and there are a variety of medications available for persons that have had a heart attack that may help to avoid a repetition. Everyone at risk should try to reduce stress in one's life or at least try to learn to cope successfully with their stressful situations.

Lung cancer kills about 150,000 people prematurely each year in the U.S. Its causes are not wholly understood but certainly genetics play a part. Also a lifetime of exposure to smoke and air contaminants increases the risk. Diets that include fruits and vegetables are thought to be helpful in avoiding this and other cancers. Articles in the popular press and nutrition publications like Prevention Magazine advocate eating fruits and vegetables such as apples, grapefruit, Brussels sprouts, broccoli and garlic. Some of these recommendations are compiled from anecdotal observations since rigorous scientific studies are difficult to conduct or interpret. That is why some recommendations change from time to time. For this reason it is a good idea to keep in touch with the latest findings on nutrition. It is expected that science will discover much more about nutrition in the years to come.

Age-related diabetes kills about 60,000 people prematurely each year in the U.S. Genetics seem to be a major part of the story here and a high blood sugar level or wounds that do not heal are early warnings. A timely diagnosis, together with proper medication and a careful diet, may enable a person with the disease to live long and well. Most doctors also recommend regular exercise.

Colo-rectal cancer kills about 50,000 people prematurely each year in the U.S. While family history is an important factor, a sedentary lifestyle together with diets high in saturated fats and red meat and low in fruits, vegetables, whole grains and beans can usually be blamed. Frequent consumption of the high-fat offerings of typical fast food restaurants seems to be a formula for colon-rectal cancer for some people in their senior years. Most doctors suggest that Third Agers should have a stool blood test every year and a Sigmoidoscopy exam every five years. Early detection may reduce the invasiveness of treatment and greatly improves the chance of survival.

Much of the same can be said to men regarding prostate cancer, the common cause of premature death among older males. Again, one should avoid diets high in fat or red meat. Many doctors recommend that senior men get a PSA (prostate specific antigen) blood test and a digital exam every year, although results are somewhat unreliable. Early detection improves chances of survival especially with the new treatment techniques. Every man over 50 should discuss his situation with his doctor annually.

For women, the big concern is breast cancer which prematurely ends the lives of 40,000 women each year in the U.S. Risk indicators include breast cancer history in mother, grandmother, aunt or sister, having a child late in life, having no children, late menopause, excessive alcohol, being overweight and having a sedentary lifestyle. Early detection often improves the chances of survival, especially with newer methods of treatment. A self-breast exam regularly in the shower or in bed and a mammogram every year should help early detection, which may prevent the need for more invasive treatment. New drugs help to retard tumor growth in some women.

The diseases mentioned above are the most common causes of premature death. There are many other less common causes such as brain tumors and a variety of other cancers. While an annual physical exam is important, the individual may be the first to recognize that something is wrong. Warning signs should not be ignored. It is far better to go to your doctor too often than too seldom.

Avoiding diseases that can be fatal is not the only concern. One should also try to avoid physical problems that can cause disability. Stroke is not only the third most common cause of death, it is also the leading cause of severe disability. A stroke happens when a blood vessel in the brain gets clogged or bursts. Depending upon what region of the brain is damaged, the effect can be loss of vision, speech, feeling, hearing or muscular control of arm, leg or face. A stroke may result in a severe headache or an immediate coma. Often there are warning signs of an impending major stroke. These symptoms are TIA's, transient ischemic attacks. They are recognized by: a sudden weakness in an arm, hand or leg; loss of feeling of one side of face or body; sudden loss of vision in one eye; loss of understanding of people talking or inability to process information; or the onset of dizziness or severe headache. If any of these symptoms occur, a doctor should be contacted immediately or call 911. The effects of TIA's are usually temporary but they are a warning that a major stroke is possible. If the carotid artery that supplies the brain with blood is plugged with fatty deposits, the risk of TIA's or stroke is increased. Some doctors may recommend that the deposits be removed surgically.

Stroke damage sometimes heals, but often the effects continue. There are stroke rehabilitation programs that can help a victim regain or develop compensating skills. The risk of stroke can be reduced if one: stops smoking, keeps blood pressure and cholesterol down, follows a low-fat diet, takes off excess weight and gets regular exercise. The American Heart Association has helpful literature on strokes. They may be contacted at 1-800-553-6321 or by writing the national center at 7272 Greenville Avenue, Dallas, TX 75231.

There are many more diseases and disorders that may not be life threatening but can greatly interfere with one's quality of life. Included are: arthritis, osteoporosis, emphysema, Alzheimer's disease and other types of dementia, clinical depression, hearing loss, migraine headaches, allergies and a variety of vision problems. Some of these conditions can be relieved with surgery, medication (including pain-relievers and anti-depressants) or devices such as walkers, hearing aids or special glasses. For some ailments, it is a matter of learning how to live with the disability and perhaps seeking professional counseling to deal with the problem. This is a vast topic that can be addressed adequately only by a team of physicians, physical therapists, speech therapists and psychologists.

To seniors suffering from painful disabilities, the credo of the Third Agers mentioned above may seem not just unrealistic but even repugnant. Although the options for disabled persons are diminished, many choices still remain. For these persons, it is suggested that they try to focus on what they can do rather than what they cannot. Those crippled with arthritis can choose activities that can be done from a comfortable chair. The whole world can be approached through reading, TV and the Internet and writing is made easier with word processors. One must be proactive in getting the newest devices to help overcome the disability. New medications offer hope and new products and technology are coming on the market every year. Frequent, shopping in drug stores and medical specialty shops may yield interesting discoveries.

Alzheimer's and stroke victims who have lost mental capability have different concerns. Their diversions have to be chosen to match their capabilities. CD-ROMs used with a computer and designed for children may provide a measure of fascination for the mentally impaired elderly. For the most part, however, they must rely on those around them for comfort and security. It is necessary for caregivers to provide physical help with daily activities, manage financial and business matters, assure the victim's safety and prevent injury, coordinate medical and rehabilitative care and provide emotional support. The disabled can help with their care by being cooperative, appreciative and cheerful with the caregiver.

When a person faces a long terminal illness, especially one that is painful or with reduced or vanished mental capability, the question of how long does a person wants to live arises. Technology has advanced to the point where a comatose person can be kept alive for years. Many people believe, as does the Hemlock Society, that when a person has totally lost the ability to communicate and has no hope of recovery, life should not be prolonged by artificial intervention. An objective that many Third Agers can support is to be healthy and functional as long as possible, but not wish for life beyond that if brain dead or in constant terminal pain.

Probably most seniors would prefer to have their final moments at home, in bed and asleep. Pneumonia with a deliriously high fever has been called "the old person's friend" because it is a relatively painless way to go. One cavalier older man once said that he would like to be shot at age 95 by his housekeeper's jealous boy friend. A curious thought, but not very realistic. Doctor-assisted "termination" is becoming more acceptable and Oregon was the first to legalize it, however, there have been few takers. One solution that has been mentioned is a "sunset cocktail"—a double martini saturated with phenobarbital. However, such a prescription is illegal in most states. Most people consider self-inflicted violence to end life to be degrading and cruel to those left behind. Some feel that it is too bad that finalizing life can't be like a graduation or wedding—planned and ceremonial.

As I write this, a woman I used to know well lies brain-dead and force-fed in a nursing home where she has resided for more than 5 years. The last time I visited her, she was not the person I knew. The form was lifeless and deformed. I do not like to remember her that way. I would not want to be remembered that way. Also, there is the cost—money that some feel might be better used for grandchildren's education or favorite charities, for example. This woman has a Living Will and Care Proxy that called for no artificial life support in case of coma and terminal illness. However, her nursing home, like many others, will not honor it for fear that some relative will object and sue. Dr. Timothy Quill, who presented the case for doctor-assisted termination to the U.S. Supreme Court in 1997, advises the preparation of a letter empowering heirs to bring suit against a nursing home or attending physician if they do not honor a valid Living Will. A copy of one's Living Will should be in the files of their primary care physician and updated every 6 or 7 years.

In that we are living longer and mostly better, a Third Age has become a magnificent opportunity for many to redefine themselves in new and interesting ways including developing one's spirituality. For those with a strong religious faith, what comes next might not be a source of anxiety. For them and others as well, there are spiritual ways of dealing with the uncertainty. We will explore these ideas in the next chapter.

"Grow old along with me, the best is yet to come.
The last of life for which the first was made."

—Elizabeth Barrett Browning

II

EXPLORING SPIRITUALITY

A Non-Religious definition of Spirituality and why it could be important to Third Agers. A View of Life after Death.

Spirituality means different things to different people. For many, it is closely associated with religious beliefs. Other views encompass the inspiration of nature, arts and the joys of family or friends. New Age religions and Zen Buddhists place much emphasis on sensitivity to an extension of inner self and senses. Meditation on these matters is their avenue to spirituality. Many find spirituality in Bible reading. Many other people think of spirituality as the inspiration they find in music, poetry, the wisdom or grace of other people, sunsets, great buildings and paintings, watching birds, trees and flowers, stars, aromas, sexual relations and even fine wine or herbal tea. Mahatma Gandhi preached that spirituality was self sacrifice and The Rev. Martin Luther King, Jr. emphasized nonviolence. In parts of the world, walking barefoot on hot coals or animal sacrifice is the way to heaven. Psychologist, Dr. C.M. Lacey, defines spirituality as a path to growing through learning.

Even clergy of a particular faith often do not agree entirely on a definition of spirituality.

The Rev. Martin Smith of the Order of St. John the Divine defines spirituality in the following ways:

It is receptivity to God.

Baptism integrates the spirit with the environment in which we live, move and have our being.

Prayer, meditation and discipline help us to experience and appreciate what we already possess.

God's spirit dwells in each individual. Spirituality is that realization.

It is knowing that God is within all people and things.

It is helping one another and seeking social justice.

It is knowing that God is in all things, not just in special places, at special times, in special people or special ceremonies.

Persons with a technical education, and very likely many others, tend to be uneasy when spiritual matters are discussed. They are more accustomed to thinking about things that can be measured, weighed or counted. They like to deal with cause and effect relationships. They prefer to describe situations with images, pictures, diagrams, or graphs. Spiritual qualities do not lend themselves very well to any of these quantitative considerations.

An alternative definition is that spirituality, in a very broad sense, consists of those qualities or facts that pertain to the spirit (or soul for some) as distinguished from physical matters. A way to define spirituality is to consider some qualities that can be described as spiritual in nature—qualities like love, courage, generosity, compassion, forgiveness, enthusiasm, loyalty and respect. Below is a supplemental list of qualities that could be called spiritual:

initiative	thoughtfulness	intelligence	humility
passion	patience	instructive	helping
integrity	kindness	consideration	diligence
dependability	leadership	creativity	beauty
honesty	cleanliness	dignity	responsibility
orderliness	grooming	advocacy	religious faith
proactivity	sharing	wisdom	cheerfulness

courtesy	pain-endurance	humor	optimism
reverence	poise	grace	enterprising
patriotism	self-reliance	sexuality	righteousness

It is obvious that none of these characteristics can be quantified beyond some qualifiers like "very" or "highly" or "memorable". It is also conceivable that every person possesses a number of these qualities to some degree, even though unquantifiable. One might say that a "profile" of a person could be defined by their prominence of these various characteristics. While the extent to which a person has these qualities is difficult to describe, salient attributes may be easy to recognize. On the other hand, these spiritual qualities are often quite personal and may not be realized at all by anyone other than the individual, who may quietly internalize the attributes.

Another attribute of a person's "spiritual profile" is that it is retained by others and can be remembered when the person is not present or might even be thousands of miles away. Moreover, the profile may be recalled, perhaps even revered, after a person has died. For many, this "spiritual profile" is a manifestation of the soul, to put the idea in a religious context.

My father had a curiosity about life after death. The night before he died, we took a walk together. He promised me that if there was life after death that he would communicate with me after he had passed on. Although more than 50 years have now gone by with nary a ghostly appearance or phone call, I am aware daily, nevertheless, of his "spiritual profile" that still influences me. In turn, I believe that I have transmitted this spirit not only to my children but, to some degree, to virtually everyone I know well. To me, this is a form of life after death. This is a perception that may appeal to others.

The computer age expression, "virtual reality", may be useful in describing a state of life after death. It fits with remembered profiles. It can be supposed that there is a state where time and location are meaningless. It can be further supposed that the spirits who dwell there are perpetually young and healthy, are never hungry, weary or in need of the things that the physical being requires. Conceivably, these spirits live on in the minds of those they touched. This is a description of the hereafter that many may find more acceptable than a vision of harp-strumming angels floating above Elysian Fields, although these and similar allegories may be a source of comfort and joy to many.

The following are excerpts from "The Art of Living Forever" by essayist, Wilfred A. Peterson:

> "No Man stands alone. Through all the centuries of recorded time, men have set in motion influences that affect your life today. You are their heir of the ages. Men reaching for the stars have created for you a world of wonder and challenge. On a more intimate note, your mother, father, teacher, clergyman, friend have built their influences into your character. More enduring than skyscrapers, bridges and cathedrals are the invisible monuments of wisdom, inspiration and example in the hearts and minds of men. Your example, your words, your ideas, your ideals can be projected into the future to live forever in the lives of others. As you throw the weight of your influence on the side of the good, the true, the beautiful, your life will achieve an endless splendor. It will go on in others, bigger, finer, nobler than you ever dared to be."

These thoughts align with the concept of a spiritual domain that is eternal. This spiritual domain pertains not only to those who are deceased, but also to those who are united spiritually who may be separated by great distances. Lovers sometimes speak of extrasensory communication. Monotheists may find spiritual joy in contemplating the thought that in something that might be called the Spiritual Domain of the Departed they will see and know God and mingle with kindred spirits.

These ideas cannot be confirmed because they deal with the unknown and unknowable, but mankind has been pondering these issues since before the dawn of history. The religions of the world can be regarded as the manifestation of these quests for knowledge looking to various prophets to make spirituality more tangible. Seemingly, Jesus understood this and made liberal use of examples, metaphors, parables and analogies to make God and the spirit understandable. Thus this book takes the position that spirituality is multi-faceted and is defined by a list of positive human qualities. It also assumes that life-after-death is a spiritual state unrelated to time and location.

If one can accept these concepts, what implication does this have for Third Agers? It can be said that in the Second Age of life, the focus of most people is on career and family. For them, the end of their physical life is probably a distant concern. Around age 60, questions about the end become more relevant. If one is going to enter a Spiritual Domain of the Departed on the best of terms, cultivation of the spirit becomes more important. In fact, for some it could be the central motivator for the remaining years of life. The Third Age, in contrast to the frantic pace and busy-ness of the First and Second Ages, provides greater opportunity to reflect upon and explore spirituality.

According to psychologist, Abraham Maslow, well known for his description of a hierarchy of needs, humans have certain prescribed physical and biological imperatives. Survival is paramount: food, clothing and shelter are commonly cited physical necessities. There are other needs not as easily understood but yet essential for human development and well-being. They include: self-esteem, security, intimacy, love of beauty, truth, sacred knowledge and the company of other people. Spirituality could be added to this list. If not a need, it could be regarded as something that would add quality to a person's life.

Effect of Spirituality on the Body

Preparing for an elevation to the Spiritual Domain of the Departed is not the only reason for exploring and developing one's spiritual qualities in the Third Age. Research sponsored by the National Institute of Health, the MacArthur Foundation and others provide mounting evidence that spirituality has an impact on physical well-being. Recent studies by Drs. Levin and Larson of the National Institute for Healthcare Research and Dr. Puchalski of George Washington School of Medicine indicate convincingly that persons with a rich spirituality and belief system do have a better record of recovery from illness and surgery. Dr. Herbert Benson of Harvard Medical School provides additional support for the idea that spirituality affects physical wellness. He describes health care as a "3-legged stool": (1) medication, (2) medical treatment including diagnostic procedures, surgery, physical and mental therapy, and (3) self-help which includes self-care along with beliefs, attitudes and coping skills. Dr. Benson asserts that an important component of self-help is spirituality. An optimistic, cheerful and loving attitude together with faith that nature will aid the curing process will, in fact, help people to get better. For many, prayer assists healing and feeling better. It wasn't long ago that this concept would have been considered unfounded conjecture by medical school faculty, although going back farther the concept was widely accepted. As cited above, mind/body interactions are becoming widely appreciated. This topic will be revisited in Chapter V.

More About Spirituality

It should be easy to realize that spirituality affects not only health, but also relationships with other people. To be convincing on this issue we only need to consider the effect projected by people who have what might be called a negative spirit. Probably all of us have known persons who are abusive, cruel, lazy, vindictive, or controlling. They may have been a neighbor, boss, co-worker or (hopefully not) one's spouse.

A list of negative spiritual attributes might also include:

gluttony	hostility	greed	hatred
selfishness	bigotry	cowardice	dishonesty
irresponsibility	envy	neglect	rudeness

In our Third Age, it seems that we are entitled to distance ourselves from people like that. It would be difficult to remember fondly people with these qualities dominating the spirit. Might a concept of "hell" be a domain dominated by the mean spirited? Most of us can quickly think of individuals with whose spirits we would not like to spend eternity.

Can spirituality be developed while excluding other people? Some would say that unless qualities like love, compassion and kindness are expressed toward others, their full potential is limited. As Mother Teresa said, "Love cannot remain by itself—it has no meaning. Love has to be put into action and that action is service". On the other hand, the strength of certain qualities like passion may exist mainly in the mind of oneself.

A personal essay could be written or contemplated about each of the spiritual qualities mentioned previously, especially if examples are considered. Each word in the list can be examined in the light of an individual's experience. Self-taught lessons in the development of spiritual qualities can be created. By thinking about each attribute, one at a time, anyone can think about how they might rate themselves and imagine how they might move to a higher level.

For example, consider the quality of courage. One can reflect on situations in his or her past when they took a risk of life or money for the sake of someone else. Was courage meritorious or deficient? What might a person have done differently if given a similar opportunity? Thinking that it's better to look forward than backward, it may be worthwhile to think about situations that may develop in the future that might be an opportunity to be courageous. One spiritual quality that warrants special consideration is love. Love includes so much and is so pervasive. There is love of spouse, family, special friends, mankind, nature, music, art, science, truth, sports, travel, literature and God. It is affection, passion, attachment, concern for others, benevolence, enduring emotional regard, charity, devotion or adoration, This list could go on. But two loves, those of God and other person(s), merit special mention. These two loves, which could be considered synonymous with honor or respect, correspond with the first two Commandments that Moses brought down off the mountain and are the basis for the laws of civilized society. God is that "higher authority" upon which our entire judicial and legal process is predicated. Without these ethics, our world would be chaos, anarchy and barbarity.

Love of God means different things to different people. It can be gratitude for the gifts of reason, memory and skill; for the talent of others and perhaps ourselves; for the magnificence of nature. It can be awe of the universe, the miracle of life and the exquisiteness of the human brain and body. It can be faith of recovery from a variety of physical or mental ills or, if we do not recover, to believe that there is something inspirational like a Spiritual Domain of the Departed that lies ahead. It can also be rejoicing in the fellowship of other people.

Love of another person has a major spiritual component that can be enormously compelling. Romantic writers, artists and musicians have been doing their best to extol love and all of its hues and variations for at least 9 thousand years. Although romance is often envisioned as the exclusive property of the young, Third Agers are not to be excluded. However, many seniors, especially those who have been married for a long time, may need a romantic boost in their love life. For love to flourish, there must be mental and emotional attraction. For those who are married, one or both of these attractions may have been eroded by years of controversy, a variety of difficulties or emotional friction. For some couples, passion burns as brightly as ever. For most, it flickers and needs refueling. For others, the flame is already out. Efforts at renewal can be rewarding.

With each passing year, the chance that one of a senior couple will soon be alone increases. He or she, along with those now single, may welcome a new love in their life. For those in search of a new attachment or those seeking to rejuvenate the old, a journey toward spiritual growth may be the pathway to a new and improved relationship. A study of one or more of Dr. Peck's books, like *The Road Less Traveled* can be inspirational.

There is another spiritual quality of special relevance to disabled Third Agers. That is the quality of pain—endurance. Pain is hardly something that people develop voluntarily, but rather have it thrust upon them. Naturally, they do what they can to relieve pain, but there may be no escape. The spirituality comes from the thoughts that one has while enduring pain. Rather than viewing one's agony in the sense of being a victim, one might better focus one's attention on the development of other spiritual qualities like charity, love and faith and reflection on the joys of life—past, present and, hopefully, the future, particularly of friends and family. For some, the empathized vision of a cross carried may be helpful and may help to overcome the anger and resentment that often accompanies a long, painful siege.

Still another quality that warrants discussion is that of reverence or religious worship. This is central to millions of peoples' spirituality. In all sects, worship is the metaphor by which spiritual imagination is defined. Every sect and denomination achieves its unique identity through its worship service. To many people, worship is the most meaningful form of spirituality. For literally billions of people around the globe, it is a magnificent experience to be within a sacred place like a cathedral or temple; hearing sacred music, liturgies, prayers and words; reading sacred Scriptures; seeing sacred objects. Even non-believers and doubters often experience a spiritual uplift when in contact with the sacred.

Spirituality, no matter how defined, can influence and interact with all that we do and think. It can be part of every issue of concern to Third Agers, even things like financial security, diet and exercise.

Consider the diagram below:

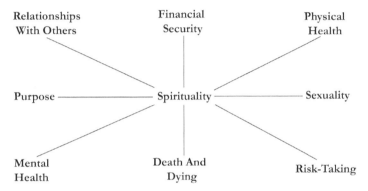

In the ensuing chapters, these issues and their interaction with spirituality will be discussed.

An important caveat must be interjected. Most of the spiritual qualities mentioned above are benevolent in nature. Unfortunately, there are countless individuals and organizations aggressively exploiting this tendency. They try to sell us products we don't need or products of inferior quality or at excessive prices (i.e.scams). They prey on our sympathies. They seem to think that all seniors are helpless, witless, irresponsible, unknowledgeable and gullible. We must show them otherwise. Be alert to high-pressure and let it be a red flag when you notice it, then exit abruptly or hang up the phone without apologies. This topic will be revisited later in the discussion of self-empowerment.

Signs of aging such as loss of hair, wrinkles, skin spots and body fat accumulations are of great concern to some seniors. Of course one can do as they feel about wigs and make-up and, as for people of all ages, good grooming and posture and attractive clothing enhances one's image and self-esteem. Think of aging looks as a medal of experience and wisdom. Here's where the glow of spirituality helps. As one senior lover said to another, "I love you and I love the package you come in, regardless." Mature observers will look beyond the loss of youthful appearance to see the substance of the person inside. For inspiration, one can recall Golda Meir, Eleanor Roosevelt and Louis Armstrong, none of whom would ever win beauty contests but who were admired for their brilliant spirits. In fact, their homeliness became a "trade mark" with worldwide recognition.

With enriched spirituality comes a joy of living, relishing each day for what it brings—the songs of birds, sunshine, rainbows, wind in the trees, the smell of grass and flowers, the beauties of waves on the shore, snow-covered mountains, beautiful music, the smile of friends, poetry, your church—whatever your neighborhood or your home has to offer. With a grand spirit, beauty is never hard to find.

Reflect, if you will, upon this Navajo prayer:

In beauty may I walk

All day long may I walk

Through the returning seasons may I walk

Beautifully birds; Beautifully joyful birds

On the trail marked with pollen may I walk

With the grasshoppers around my feet may I walk

With dew about my feet may I walk

With beauty behind me may I walk

With beauty above me may I walk

With beauty all around me may I walk

In old age wandering on a trail of beauty, living again may I walk

It is finished in beauty.

III

A Vision of Enjoyment, Reward, Fulfillment and Purposeful Options in Your Third Age

Now is the time for reaping the rewards of a productive life; a time for study, travel, recreation and hobbies; a time for Spiritual Eldering especially for grandchildren. Now is an opportunity to develop your own spirituality by doing for others—volunteer work, family caregiving, teaching, writing family history; to reaffirm your religious faith. Hopefully, a chance to do what you've always wanted or meant to do

I have two former friends who approached their retirement in what I would judge to be unfortunate ways. When I asked one how he was spending his retirement, he answered "I sit and do crossword puzzles until the mail arrives" The other stayed in bed until 10am then arose, made a pitcher of martinis and spent the rest of the day watching soap operas on television. Both died in their mid-60's. Is there a lesson to be learned?

Whenever a retiree says to me "I've paid my dues, I'm going to take it easy now", I think of my two deceased friends. I share a belief with others that the key to a fruitful Third Age is being useful to someone, some cause, somehow as long as you live. This book champions that message.

Some individuals have had careers that provided great personal importance, influence, prestige and rewards. For them, the adjustment to retirement may be difficult. In that regard, I think of Frank and Jean who left Chicago, where he had been an aggressive president of a large company, and moved to Phoenix to avoid winter chill and enjoy lots of golf. He knew a few people in Phoenix and expected that his reputation and former influence would provide them with an instant circle of friends. It was harder than he had expected. They joined a golf club and met a number of people but admission to their established "circles" proved to be elusive. After three years of trying to command a court of admirers with scant success, Frank and Jean gave up and moved to La Jolla where he thought he might find better contacts. The welcoming committee never came. Still another move to Carmel produced the same result. Frank and Jean now live in Palm Springs still intently trying to reconstruct a power base instead of extending themselves graciously to others in an appealing way.

Another acquaintance, David, spent a career with a large company in a position that was important and financially rewarding, but spiritually deadening. In retirement, he moved to Maine to be near his beloved seacoast. Instead of just watching the ocean, he began to build model boats. He contacted an area boat builder and started making miniatures of their cruising sailboats that were sold to wealthy customers for $400,000 and up. David makes exact, beautifully-crafted models of these boats for about $5,000 each. From the point of view of a customer who is spending a half million or so for his boat, what's another $5000 for a model to be displayed in the office or den? David makes one of these in his basement shop in about 40 hours and turns out about one per month. It is not only a nice income supplement but a chance to be spiritually uplifted by being intimate with these gorgeous sailing craft. It is a joy he never experienced on his job.

Some retirees call it a second chance. Others call it a godsend. It's the moment when they discover—or stumble upon—what they were probably always meant or wanted to do with their lives. And now they are doing it. But it's not always easy to plan. It's often a matter of discovery. It may take several tries to find the right thing. A formula that has been successful for many is to be proactive in a variety of ways and let serendipity happen. Several hooks on the line make catching a fish more likely.

All of this has special relevance if one is contemplating a move to a new community to enjoy a better climate or mountain or ocean views. It is wise to try out a new area first as a tourist studying churches and clubs that can be a vehicle for finding new friends. Perhaps a long trip via RV visiting many prospective communities is a good method for some to scope out the possibilities.

Who says it's too late to start over with a new beginning? Consider the fact that Geothe completed Faust at age 80, Titian was painting masterpieces at 98; Toscanini was still conducting at 85; Edison was busy in his laboratory at 84 and Benjamin Franklin was helping to frame the American Constitution at 80. Note also that Jack Lemmon, Paul Newman, Walter Matthau and Frank Sinatra have been box office stars well beyond age 70. Ann Landers and Mike Wallace are still going strong at 80 plus. What more can be said about John Glenn who undertook a second voyage in space at age 77?

Of course very few Third Agers will become world famous, but there are numerous lesser but noble endeavors that are within the realm of possibility for almost all. The supreme joy of the Third Age is the marvelous array of choices that are available.

Options.

For the benefit of those individuals who are approaching retirement or are newly retired, a review of a list of retirement activity options may be useful. The list may also be helpful for those who are restless or feeling unfulfilled in retirement, for ongoing homemakers observing an apparently aimless retired spouse or for those who may be developing programs for retirees. The "menu" below lists a number of options. Scanning this list may suggest some possibilities to those who don't already have a firm idea of what they want to do in their Third Age.

Anyone can expand this list. It is offered as a starting point in Third Age planning. However, it has been said that life is what happens when you are planning something else. In other words, one might begin participation in a new activity that turns out not to be an end in itself but a pathway that leads to something else that's a better fit with one's interests. Make a start and let the unexpected happen.

How might these ideas relate to one's spirituality? The thought is offered that spiritual development might be a primary goal in the Third Age and that activities like those in the "menu" can provide the pathway to a greater fulfillment.

A "Menu" Of Retirement Activitiy Options

For **Recreation** there is tennis, golf, swimming, all kinds of travel, hiking, bowling, biking, skiing, hunting, fishing, boating, flying, many different card and board games, dancing, puzzle working, nature walking, etc.

One can **Study** literature, music, art, religion, languages, science, computer, other cultures, gerontology, and much more at a local university or senior organization like OASIS. One can complete an (additional) academic degree.

One can seek **Employment** full time or part time. If trained and experienced, one can do consulting, writing or teaching. One can start up or invest in and be active in a small business.

Grandparenting can be a consuming activity teaching, coaching and entertaining grandchildren and other children.

Devote time to **Hobbies** such as photography, model building, sewing, cooking, collecting, genealogy, playing of piano or other musical instrument in a group or alone, painting, home improvement, stock market, woodworking, winemaking.

The world needs **Volunteers** for administering and supporting almost every non-profit organization from museums to Red Cross, Salvation Army and numerous support groups for victims of diseases and their families. All need help with fund raising and publicity. There are a huge variety of community service opportunities such as service to disadvantaged, church or volunteer ambulance duty, literacy education, Rotary, Compeer and Habitat for Humanity.

Although **Caregiving** and service to family and friends in need may be more of an imperative than an option for many, it is a voluntary gesture of love for others. That surely is true in the case of pets.

Political Action needs helpers for mailing, campaigning, fund raising, and getting out voters. Many seniors run for office. If they win, they have the opportunity to serve the public through better government.

Making new friends is a challenge to be met if one moves to a new community or loses a spouse or partner. One needs to be enterprising. Ways to do this include joining discussion or special interest groups and being visible and proactive.

A **Mentor** assists young people with personal problem solving or professional advancement or one may serve in an organization like SCORE (Service Corps Of Retired Executives).

All **Charities** need supporters to donate money or the equivalent in services.

By **Networking** one can facilitate communication among family members and friends.

Family Archives and history need to be documented and preserved.

Finally there's **Enjoyment**—old-fashioned rest and relaxation and, of course, dining out, theatre, TV, movies, Internet and reading for pleasure.

Pursuing the thought of letting a personal goal of spiritual development guide the selection of retirement activity options, some specific comments are made below.

Recreation

Many seniors were devotees of golf, fishing or card games in their Second Age and regard retirement as the time when they can enjoy endless pursuit of their passion. Others may look upon retirement as a time to take up or focus more on various kinds of recreational activities.

Can golf really be a spiritual activity? Many golfers return home angry and frustrated and showing symptoms of too much time at the 19th hole. Is this spiritual? Well, when one considers the fact that golf was invented by Presbyterians, it is likely that it was never intended to be enjoyable, but instead to be a "character builder". However, golf can be spiritual if one enjoys the scenic beauties of the course, good fellowship that can go with the game, the quest for perfection and an exercise in humility. On the other hand, if the game becomes a license for display of anger, arrogance, extravagant spending, neglect of home life or obnoxious behavior (all of which have been witnessed), any spiritual value (and very likely good performance) has been lost.

On the plus side, personal contacts made in the clubhouse may be the way to discovering unexpected avenues of personal fulfillment. Opportunities sometimes come from unexpected sources. However, not all options that come to a person are beneficial, so one has to discriminate by asking "will this opportunity enhance my personal fulfillment and spirituality or will it not". If not, pass it up and wait for something better to happen or come along.

How about tennis as a sport for Third Agers? It has been said that the best way to keep an aging brain functioning well is to have an activity that combines a physical and mental challenge. Tennis seems to fill this bill quite well. What's more, it should be noted that tennis was invented by Anglicans who probably figured that line calls were a test of truth-fulness and concomitant character analysis. Bridge, too, is mentally challenging and many find it a way to stay alert and cunning. However, there is little physical exercise in bridge unless one kicks their partner a lot under the table.

Unfortunately, tennis is not for those with hip, knee or foot disabilities. For them, there are alternatives like canoeing or rowing, both of which can be very pleasurable exercise for those who live near water. Bicycling can be enjoyed by people with mild leg disabilities since there is little knee impact and body weight is supported. Of course for many people, especially those who never did enjoy strenuous physical activities, none of the above may be appealing. Also, there are those with other disabilities that may preclude many physical recreational activities. However, numerous seniors find satisfaction in just plain walking—in the neighborhood, in parks or in shopping malls. Those with considerable disability can still exercise in pools, dance in place or seated or do isometric exercises (Muscle flexing without movement).

Many men and a few women are ardent hunters. Is there a spiritual component to hunting? Can man love animals and yet kill them? One can rationalize hunting by noting that humans are innately carnivorous and, while vegetarians seem to function well without meat in their diets, most people prefer their protein in the form of animal products. Presuming that animals must be killed in order for man to eat meat, hunters make no apologies for their sport. Personally, I love steak, chops and Big Macs occasionally, but don't ask me to perform the killing. I think it may be redeeming, however, to read the following by hunter-writer, Jimmy Rolinson:

The canvasback is the king of ducks in the old hunter's book and an epicure's delight in the bargain. He is the hardest of them all to hit as he hurtles hell-bent across the sky. The big bulls remind you of a jet fighter with their bullet heads and short, small, swept-back wings. Those wings claw air at such a furious clip that they send their big, fat bodies racing along faster than any duck. They are straightaway speed-sters made for a big track, and they never flare or dodge.

Fishermen have sincere feelings as expressed in their bumper stickers: "A bad day fishing is better than a good day at work" and "Each day spent fishing is a day's addition to one's lifespan".

These are sportsmen's views of spiritual enrichment. However, I fully realize that many people are opposed to the killing of animals and may find these ideas distasteful and I empathize with them.

With regard to travel, it removes a person from his or her tight home setting and transports one's thoughts as well as person to a new milieu making one a more worldly citizen. Travel can make one appreciative of other regions and cultures; knowledgeable of the geography, history, tradition, art and architecture of other countries and places; an ambassador of good will; and better informed regarding global issues. Travel can be so personally compelling that many people define them-selves in terms of their travels. I suggest that one should travel with the objective of spiritual enhancement through seeing the beauty of other parts of the world and understanding different cultures and being awed by nature. For those who are fond of these experiences, there are never enough opportunities. But not all travel is easy and pleasant, in fact, it can be a miserable experience for those who have a fear of flying or a low tolerance for unexpected delays, unfamiliar languages or are uncomfortable in alien surroundings. Still others may worry about getting sick in a foreign country. Some people would simply rather be comfortable at home. This can become a thorny issue among couples where one person likes to travel and the other doesn't. Travel groups and clubs make single travel easier and safer and many married couples separate for a while to go on trips the other might not enjoy. Furthermore, separation in these cases provides a temporary opportunity for "stretch out" space which some marriages need.

Study

Thinking back to your high-school days, you may recall that some guidance counselors advised young people not to major in subjects like fine arts or European history in college because there were few jobs in these fields. Instead, the counselors would suggest that, if people found these and similar non-vocational subjects especially interesting, they should pursue them on their own time or in retirement. For Third Agers, that time is NOW. These are the years in which to read the classics as well as current best sellers. It's also a great opportunity to visit art galleries, attend concerts and theatre, get in touch with your chosen religion, learn a second (third, fourth or fifth) language, become computer literate, catch up with science and medicine, complete or get another degree and understand gerontology.

Many colleges offer non-credit courses for seniors at reduced rates. Many communities have senior citizen groups that offer educational tours. OASIS (Older Adult Service and Information System) offers short Courses in subjects of interest to seniors. OASIS has facilities in most major cities. Elderhostel specializes in educational travel for seniors. Their quarterly catalog is very large. Their publication states: Elderhostel is a non-profit organization committed to being the pre-eminent provider of high quality, affordable, educational opportunities for older adults. We believe learning is a lifelong process. Sharing new ideas, challenges and experiences is rewarding in every season of life. Elderhostel can be contacted at 75 Federal Street, Boston, MA 02110-1941.

Employment

The suggestion that a senior take on a full or part-time job for pay may seem incongruous or even offensive for some retirees. For others, it may offer a special opportunity. Gainful employment can provide a sense of usefulness that can boost self-esteem. A regular job can keep one challenged and alert, may keep old skills current, or put one in touch with other people. For many, the money may be important in meeting expenses. One might work in his or her own field of expertise on salary, by the project or as a contract consultant. On the other hand, one can do something entirely different from their former profession or trade. If one likes to write, local newspapers may find your skills valuable. Teaching part-time in places like museums or being a tour guide are other options. Of course, working may make more sense for some than others for physical reasons.

Retirees often start or buy small businesses such as gift shops or run a "Bed and Breakfast" in a resort area. However, caution is advised. Many such ventures fail financially washing away the badly needed life savings of the retiree. Furthermore, the workweek can be very lengthy. That can be miserable, especially if the effort is losing money. Beware of ego trips and confusing a hobby with a business. Before starting any venture, always calculate the cash flow over the first few years by estimating income pessimistically and estimating expenses with allowance for unpleasant surprises to see how bad the negative cash flow can get. Can you stand it financially and psychically?

If you are fortunate enough to afford money for speculation, You can consider investment, with or without working, in a new venture started by a smart, young, energetic guy with no money. Look for these opportunities through the local newspaper or, better yet, through trustworthy contacts. Many small businesses have been started this way, but not all succeed. Beware of zealots in love with their idea but out of touch with reality. Go through the cash flow exercise with skepticism. A few old geezers in Silicon Valley and elsewhere have made (second) fortunes this way. Others wish they'd never heard of the idea.

Grandparenting

Rabbi Schlacter-Shalomi, founder of the Spiritual Eldering Institute, regards grandparenting as the most important activity in which a senior can engage. Here is what he says: "Why should anyone live longer than the time of begetting and raising our children? If we do live longer, then nature must have some kind of purpose. The purpose is to house consciousness for generation to generation so that the older generation can transmit something to the younger."

Otherwise stated, one may recognize the need to transmit traditional values to the grandchildren. Those of us who are in our 70's grew up in the 1930's when work was considered good fortune, pleasures were comparatively simple, law was respected, patriotism was fairly universal, honesty prevailed and many children became Boy or Girl Scouts. Our children probably grew up in the 1950's and 60's—the Woodstock generation—where authority was defied, work was to be avoided and patriotism was considered chauvinistic. TV violence and sexual permissiveness were commonplace. Grandparenting is an opportunity to pass on the values and customs in which we believe. Also, for many of us, our possessions and whatever wealth we may have might eventually pass to our grandchildren and we want to prepare them to receive it and take care of it.

Bonding with the grandchildren is necessary to achieve these objectives. This is not always easy, especially if they live far away. Even if they live nearby, some special techniques are needed to make the bonding work. Here are some thoughts:

1. Make bonding enjoyable. Do together the things that the child likes. Be patient and tolerant of messes and noise.

2. Give a guided tour of your home. Point out prize possessions, especially those with family significance, and photographs.

3. Demonstrate exemplary behavior and manners, but do not be preachy. Talk about caring for others, property and the environment. Coach them on how to endear themselves to others.

4. Be a good story teller—provide humorous stories of your youth, their parents, your parents, your travels.

5. Read aloud to young children.

6. Play games or take them hiking, boating, swimming, skiing, bowling; take them to sports events; to concerts. Magic tricks are long-remembered. Present the unique features of your town.

7. Spend as much time as possible with them year after year as they grow. Travel to them if they can't get to you conveniently .

8. Take advantage of the fact that working parents need a break and invite the children to stay with you, or you might go to take care of them, while the parents are away. However, enforce the limits agreed to with their parents regarding hours and activities.

9. Give them small, thoughtful gifts. Expensive gifts and money... may not offer any more pleasure or enjoyment to them when they are youngsters. Teenagers, however, begin to appreciate monetary tokens, especially cash, to purchase items of their own choosing.

10. Talk about careers and education. Offer tutoring, if needed.

If you have no grandchildren, grand nieces and nephews or even unrelated or neglected children (of which there are many) may welcome your attention.

Hobbies

The array of hobbies available to seniors is myriad. Hobbies can have a spiritual component if they preserve something rare, result in a display that entertains or educates other people or provides a service or useful object to others as well as one's self.

Photography, for example, can preserve images of people and places for "the times of our life". Photos can entertain viewers regarding one's travels, treating others to beauties that they may not have known. A collection of photographs taken over a long time period and attractively displayed is an excellent memorial for the dearly departed.

Woodworking, sewing and other crafts may carry an unforgettable message of love while providing fine gifts for friends and family. Gourmet, or at least thoughtful, cooking for others is an act of spiritual giving. Though the dinner is gone with the washing of the dishes, the meal may be memorable if presented as a token of friendship or love in an atmosphere of conviviality.

Some collections are truly valuable jewelry, antiques, dolls, coins, stamps, rare books, art works or other interesting bric-a-brac. Not only can the assembly of some collections be quite exhilarating for the collector, but also the collection may have spiritual and sentimental value if the objects have been acquired with the supplementary thought of passing along to heirs something of special value. In fact, if one has an heir or friend that admires one of your collected objects, consider giving it away now rather than "later".

Compiling family archives is a very important activity for seniors and, hopefully, there is someone in every family who has an interest in genealogy. Family trees are hard to construct if starting from a base of zero. Unless the information has been captured by the previous generation, most people would not know who their great-grandparents were or where and how they lived and died.

Opportunities for seniors with musical or performing talents or interests abound in most communities. For example, New Horizons is a musical organization that consists of retirees who are reviving their instrumental skills. They perform for community organizations and for their own enjoyment as well as that of their audiences. New Horizon bands have been organized in many cities including: Carefree, AZ; Charlottesville, VA; Davenport, IA; Eugene, OR; Hagerstown, MD; Hartford, CT; Indianapolis, IN; Iowa City, IA; La Cruces, NM; Loveland, CO; Madison, WI; Milwaukee. WI; Rochester, NY; Santa Barbara, CA; Tacoma, WA; Winnetka, IL; Wichita, KS; and Winston-Salem, NC. Other opportunities for musical production, singing groups and amateur theatre or dance troupes are found in many places. One should check the local newspaper for either want-ads or notice of performances to find contacts.

Volunteering

Volunteer options are countless and varied. Volunteers can donate their time, energy and talent to causes they value. Many non-profit organizations depend on volunteers to function and for many volunteers it almost becomes full-time employment (without getting paid). Those who serve may feel that they are compensated by the satisfaction they derive from making the world a better place in which to live. Third Agers, as a group, make an enormous contribution to the country as a result of their volunteer efforts.

The opportunities for meaningful service abound. Every museum, every church, every hospital, almost every office of every nonprofit organization counts on the efforts of volunteers. Add to that the Red Cross, volunteer ambulance and fire-fighting service, hiking trail maintenance, Rotary, Habitat for Humanity, U.S. Power Squadron and many others. If there is a medical or emotional problem in a family, a support group probably exists locally to provide information and coping skills consultation regarding the disorder. These groups are seeking to involve participants who, by helping others, help themselves. Also, most non-profit organizations have a great need for volunteers to assist in fundraising—not always enjoyable, but very necessary.

Other very meaningful volunteer jobs include museum docent, teacher's assistant, Sunday School teaching, and literacy training for immigrants, to name just a few. Usually, one phone call to an agency brings engagement. To the extent that they may have benefited from the activities of non-profit organizations, **able** retirees with discretionary time may feel an obligation to provide volunteer service. Above all, volunteering is almost always a learning and "feel good" experience.

Caregiving

In the words above, volunteer efforts were encouraged for those who are able. Some people simply are not able because of their own disabilities or those for whom they have a caregiving responsibility. An ill spouse or close friend or relative may require constant attention. Seldom is this responsibility welcome, but once the problem is evident, care-giving duties are likely to take precedence over almost everything else. Many caregivers find that the responsibility can be all-consuming, especially if the person cared for is bed-bound and would be better off in a nursing home if the family could afford the cost. A common problem one finds today is that of a 70-year-old son or daughter or son needing care him or herself while also having the responsibility of caring for a 95-year-old parent.

There may be few pleasures that come the way of isolated caregivers. Television and other forms of home entertainment help to relieve the tedium. Pen pals or chat room friends found on the Internet can bring some relief and joy to an otherwise dismal life.

Two Internet references are:

Companion Express at www.companionex@aol.com and Senior-Site at www.senior-site.com

In many communities, a respite service is available to enable caregivers to travel or pursue interests outside the home.

Pets, particularly a dog or cat, can provide an emotional boost and companionship to those who are cut off from normal social contacts. In many ways, animals may be easier to get along with than impatient caregivers. Research has indicated that pet owners may live longer as a result of the nurturing that a pet owner gives and receives from the dog or cat.

There is one unpleasant caveat—beware of elder abuse. Disabled elders can be victims of the greed, impatience and/or anger of unwilling or stressed caregivers. If there is such a threat, other family members should be notified or one can call Lifeline or other local abuse hot lines for help,

Politics

In spite of frequent negative perceptions, politics are the essence of democracy. "Good politicians" can be defined as ones with good moral character who listen to their constituents and vote on issues that respect supporters' wishes that are consistent with the good of the majority of people. If we want to have an elective government, every one who can should be involved in the process. The procedure for selection of candidates usually is reserved for those who have helped the party by volunteering in mailing, polling, publicity and fund raising. To be a candidate, it is even more essential to have participated as a volunteer or as a fund donor or both. Third Agers are often the ones best able to contribute time and money and even run for office, as did my friend, Van, who at age 68 was elected to our County Legislature. Since he was financially secure and didn't need to worry about reelection, Van would speak and vote his conscience and not worry about "political correctness". A courageous person like that is badly needed amid cautious party liners.

Is there a spiritual component to politics? If we want decent people in government, people with integrity need to get involved and attract similar types of people to the process. Far too many candidates are motivated by the thrill of power or influence or maybe even the possibility of monetary kickbacks or other types of largess. While it is unrealistic to expect politicians to be totally selfless servants of the people, their highest priority ought to be their desire to contribute to good government.

In a democracy, it is to be expected that the political process will include many types of extremist minorities, some with religious affiliations, with an agenda they wish to impose on the majority. A plurality of level-headed, fair-minded politicians is needed to have sensible government. Honest, sincere, intelligent, balanced Third Agers are needed to protect the country from any vocal minority of one-issue zealots. If you aren't able to participate in the process, at least vote. Seniors can make a lot of difference. Their votes count.

Making New Friends

Old friends are wonderful since in their mind's eyes, you are still young. They may remember when your children were born and when you got your new 1953 Chevrolet and the 2-family picnics you enjoyed together way back when. However, one of the great joys of the Third Age can be making new friends in new situations.

We know that many seniors choose or find it necessary to move to a new and unfamiliar location. Many desire to move to a warmer climate, from the city to the country or to a resort area, from the country to the city, from flat prairie to mountains or seashores or somewhere closer to a son or daughter. Many also wish to downsize from a multi-bedroom house that was great for raising a family to something easier and less costly to maintain, and often in a totally new community. Maybe it's time for a retirement home. Sooner or later, all couples are separated and the survivor must learn to function as a single person perhaps in a new surrounding. In all of these situations, making new friends and acquaintances is an important skill.

What are friends for? For seniors, perhaps the most important reason is that friends are a support system—persons who know you and would notice if you have a problem and be ready to help. They are people who care about you,remember your birthday and your favorite taste treat and are concerned about any health problems you might have. Included are people who are interested in your past career and adventures, your children and what you have to say. Friends also are important for a healthy mind and that can help body wellness. It almost goes without saying that if one is to have friends, one must be a friend to others.

Here are seven suggestions for making friends in a new situation.

1. Be visible. Walk the neighborhood. Dress attractively. If you have a dog, let him help you meet other dog owners (but don't let him foul the neighbor's lawn). Wave to neighbors from your car even if you don't know them.

2. Be a volunteer. What better way to meet other volunteers. Looking for friends. Join discussion groups at church or senior citizen groups.

3. Be proactive. Invite prospective friends for coffee, for a drink, for dinner or to go to the theatre. Single women seeking male companionship need to realize that it's OK to take the initiative.

4. Smile often. Make yourself attractive. If gravitational pull on facial fat has taken its toll over the years and made your smile look more like a sardonic grimace, perhaps an investment in cosmetic surgery is warranted.

5. Be cheerful. Minimize complaints. Don't use friends as an "emotional dumping ground" unloading all your grievances on the unwary. Try to put a positive "spin" on life; avoid dispensing gloomy thoughts.

6. Think of making new friends as a spiritual adventure. Be interested in what they have to say. Look for opportunities to distribute compliments sincerely and often, even for minor things.

7. Avoid being the purveyor of negative information about others (i.e. gossip). Savvy seniors are quick to recognize the threat of reciprocity.

Loneliness is the toxic substance of the Third Age. Loneliness often begets more loneliness because the lonely person often tends to be bitter and self-pitying, inward and uncaring about others. The solution to the problem is to be proactive in seeking out other people employing the suggestions above. Friend-seeking need not be in-person. One can use the telephone or even e-mail or Internet. New friends can make the Third Age the best ever.

Mentoring

Something Third Agers can often do well is to help young people advance in their careers and improve their lives by passing along the fruits of one's experience. During his working years, a man who was a company officer, manager or senior professional or craftsman, could see to it that promising young subordinates were given special opportunities to gain valuable insight and experience and develop access to an old-boy network that would help them move upward. Although the old power base of influence probably has eroded for most retirees, one may still have much valuable advice to give—mostly in the form of caveats—what not to do. Experience may be a euphemism for our mistakes in life and, if you can keep young people from making mistakes in judgement, you've done them a great service.

The situation of elder women mentoring a young lady is somewhat different. Many elder women can help young women in the same business or professional way as men, but also they can be helpful as a source of child raising information or family problem-healing advice or useful social introductions.

However, one might be aware that many young people are not fond of seeking advice from geriatrics, especially their parents. Some will ask for advice and it's far better if that happens spontaneously rather than making an offer that is spurned. As young people mature, they may seek a "partnership" on a project. Be ready to help. Even though one may be highly capable of offering good advice, don't be surprised if there are no takers.

The English have an organization called "Dark Horse" which offers mentoring by seniors without obligation. Also there is the International Executive Service Corps (IESC), an organization of retired executives and professionals that provide volunteer consulting services to fledgling businesses in developing countries. IESC may be contacted at Box 10005, Stamford, CT 06904.

Charitable Giving

If one is fortunate enough to have accumulated wealth beyond his or her foreseeable needs, it is probably unwise to retain it to the end because inheritance taxes may take away a large portion of the assets. It is better to spend surplus money or give it away while one is living for several reasons. Significant wealth is difficult to spend without waste. There is a limit to what one can eat or drink. A large house or houses, yacht or stable of horses are a management and maintenance burden. Travel can be stressful and uncomfortable. With art works and other precious collections, there is the constant worry of theft or destruction.

By contrast, wealth can benefit mankind and bring a huge spiritual uplift if used to support a favorite charity—a school, hospital, medical research laboratory, church or other non-profit organization. Rather than spread gifts to many organizations, it may be most satisfying to focus on one or two so that a significant impact can be witnessed. College dormitories, hospital wings, libraries and other private facilities across the country bear the names of generous people who felt that way.

For those of lesser but still sizable means, a form of philanthropy that has become increasingly popular is the Charitable Gift Annuity. If one owns stock or other asset with considerable capital appreciation, one can transfer the stock to a participating charity of choice and receive in return a tax deduction and income for life. Typically, appreciated stock yields little in the way of dividends, whereas the income from the trust fund that the charity operates usually yields much more. The donor receives both increased income and a charitable tax deduction. When the donor dies, the stock is not part of the estate subject to inheritance tax.

A memorial gift that represents thankfulness for the life of a deceased friend directed to the charity that would have been the departed person's choice benefits the donor as well as the recipient.

Family Networking

A very important function that an energetic grandparent can provide is to be the center of a communication network for the whole family. One can imagine a dozen grandchildren scattered all over the globe wondering about each other—weddings, births, jobs, illnesses, etc. If they all send grandma(pa) a brief note via e-mail each month, (s)he can forward copies to all others with minimum effort adding appropriate comments. All this is possible by regular mail, but e-mail makes it vastly easier, quicker and less expensive. No big family should be without e-mail if they can afford it. "Set-top boxes" that play through the TV and do only e-mail and Internet are both inexpensive and very easy to use.

Family Archives

A project of considerable value and pleasure for all grandparents to consider is to construct a family tree and write a family history for distribution to all descendants. It leaves the future generation with a legacy of both identity and love. The grandchildren may not be interested now, but they probably will be later in life. People tend to start taking an interest in these matters about age 50. It can be a formidable task, especially for large families, but if it is not done, some vital information may be lost forever.

Here are three suggestion regarding how to go about it.

1. For you and your spouse, identify all of your grandparents—their names, the dates of their life span, where they were born, where they lived, what they did and where they are buried.

2. Create four "tree" diagrams showing all the descendants for each pair of grandparents. Compile the same information (dates and places) for each person in the tree. At this point, things start to get complicated and it is advisable to give each descendant an "identification number" to reference a paragraph describing their life. For those who have died, it is well to note the cause of death for future genetic intelligence.

3. For each grandchild, create a diagram that shows each of his or her parents, grandparents, great-grandparents, great-great-grandparents and so forth as far back as you can go.

If you do not presently have all this information, there are various sources that can help. For persons born in the U.S., the Church of Jesus Christ of Latter Day Saints (i.e. the Mormon Church) in Salt Lake City is probably the best single source of family records available. They can be contacted at any of their local Family History Centers (tm) or call 1-800-346-6044. Birth, death and marriage records in resident cities or towns are also good sources. If you cannot find the information you need to complete the family story, do the best you can.

Family histories are made far more interesting if accompanied by photos. Pictures of homes and individuals at various stages of life add a lot. Photos can be laid out several to a page with captions added and duplicated with a color copier. Combine that with a narrative describing interesting facts and anecdotes regarding key family members and the whole is a very nice package. Duplicated and bound by a local copy shop, the family history is a document that will be appreciated for a long time, maybe centuries. With a little more effort, the whole work, pictures and all can be scanned and placed on a compact disk (CD) for even greater archival preservation. Your "spirit" gracing the work will give you another kind of eternal life. Think about that!

Enjoyment

Many retirees consider that this is what the Third Age is all about—to enjoy life—to kick back and smell the roses. On the other hand, there are some newly retired persons who attack their newfound freedom with frantic exuberance and take on so many activities that they create a stressful situation for not only themselves but also those around them. Life may become very difficult for a spouse who is not so motivated. Those who believe that retirement is meant to be total comfortable relaxation are so entitled provided it is not an imposition on those close to them. This brings us to the issue of spousal conflict.

Spousal Conflict Resolution

In retirement, husband and wife may be in closer proximity for more time than ever before and the characteristics of one that might have been slightly bothersome before may now become major irritants. One's being too busy or too lazy in the judgement of the other can be a source of difficulty in the marriage. Similarly, the interests of one spouse may not be shared by the other. A compromise or resolution should be negotiated if the relationship is to be harmonious. The critical spouse needs to develop his/her own interests or challenges and should avoid trying to control or "micro-manage" the other. Family counselor and lecturer, Dr. C. Marrett Lacey, suggests that the best relationships appear to be ones in which a partner who does not share a particular interest agreeably suggests "why don't you go alone or with friends". In that way, no one feels imposed upon. Group counseling is popular among many retiree groups. They recognize that often needs and values change in the Third Age and relationships may need a re-evaluation. Ultimatums like "I'll go if you go" are not constructive. The pursuit of a more satisfactory life has to have individual "buy-in" for a lasting success.

A resolution of spousal conflicts may involve a reallocation or prioritization of time—less volunteer time and more time with the partner dining out, reading, listening to music, theatre and restful travel—activities of mutual enjoyment. Appeasement of one member of a couple to calm the other is likely to have only temporary value. Both need to be free to select their favored activities. In any event, there must be time for communication and discussion of differences. Suffering in silence is not a satisfactory solution. Even if a couple has been married for many years, a change in situation can precipitate new stresses and the services of a marriage counselor may be very useful if group counseling is unavailable or unsatisfactory.

This section of this book has been a reminder of quite a few options for Third Age activities. There are many more possibilities. An in-depth source of ideas is provided by OASIS (Older Adult Services & Information Services) chapters of which are located in most major cities. They provide short courses in arts, humanity, wellness, practical living, travel and more. The OASIS Institute central office is located at this time at 7710 Carondelet Avenue, St. Louis, MO 63105; phone 314-662-2149.

Again, it is suggested that one's spiritual development should be the central criterion for selecting options. This approach is offered as a basis for a more satisfying Third Age of life.

The following is an adaptation of a quote from philosopher, Samuel Ullman, that expresses this thought:

"Youth is not a time of life; it is a state of mind. It is not a matter of rosy cheeks, red lips and supple knees; it is a matter of the will, a quality of the imagination, a vigor of the emotions; it is the freshness of the deep springs of life. Youth means the predominance of courage over timidity, of the appetite for adventure over the love of ease. This often exists in a man of 60 more than a boy of 20. Nobody grows old merely by a number of years. We grow old by deserting our ideals. Years may wrinkle the skin, but to give up enthusiasm wrinkles the soul. Worry, fear, self-distrust bows the heart and turns the spirit to dust. Whether 70 or 17, there is in every human being's heart the lure of wonder, the unfailing child-like appetite for what's next and the joy of the game of living. In your heart there is a radio receiver; so long as it receives messages of beauty, hope, cheer and courage, you are young. When your spirit is covered with the snows of cynicism and the ice of pessimism, then you have grown old, even at 20. But as long as your radio receives messages of optimism, there is hope that you may die young at 90."

IV

REALIZING FINANCIAL COMFORT AND SECURITY IN YOUR THIRD AGE

Ideas for: Managing Expenses to Match Resources; Investment Management Now and "Forever"; taking Distribution of your 401(k) or IRA; Charitable Gift Annuities to have your Financial Cake and Eat It too; Living Trusts; Pre Nuptial Agreements and Risk Management for Seniors.

A common complaint among seniors is, "I wish I had earned and/or saved more when I was working". Although after age 65 is a little late to improve one's fortunes, the situation need not be all that discouraging. In the first place, how much money does a person really need? A flippant answer might be, "20% more than they have". By and large, it's hard for most retirees to increase their income very much. The main strategy for seniors is to try to live within their means. However, with uncertainties galore, living within income may be difficult for many people, especially if they live longer than they expected or encounter chronic health problems and if inflation is worse than expected.

If we only knew exactly how long we would live, we could crank through some computer program that would tell us just how long our money (income plus reserves) would last and then die the day our last dollar is gone. By spending less we would give our heirs the fun of our money rather than ourselves (which may be a choice for some). To spend more would eventually wipe out reserves and force still lower spending or maybe even make one dependent upon family or welfare. Not long ago, being dependent on family in one's old age was the common plan for many. In view of Social Security and other retirement income plans, fewer families are expecting to care for their aging parents and might not do it cheerfully. Most Third Agers need to anticipate self support to the end, if possible.

Self-support should start with a financial plan. Some may need the help of a professional planner. Financial planners usually start a plan by asking questions around the costs of food, shelter, clothing, transportation and other essentials, gradually building to some minimum total financial requirement year by year to expected longevity. Perhaps without asking about gifts, travel or luxuries, the typical planner may find a financial surplus on paper with which they will try to sell one of their "products"—life insurance, mutual funds, real estate partnerships or the like or maybe long term health care insurance. Their advice may be optimum, but one should always be suspect when it is realized that a sales commission "is part of the solution." A second or third opinion from a different advisor and/or an estate-planning lawyer is worth seeking before signing any contract.

People fortunate enough to have ample income and/or investments might approach things in a different way. They may not have to worry a great deal about budgeting for utility bills, food or car insurance. Enough money for essentials is always there. They can focus instead on major options like travel, new cars, house redecoration, charity, gifts to children and grandchildren or new investments. For these people, budgets don't make much sense. If things get tight, they simply postpone the next trip or make it closer to home or of shorter duration or trim back gifts to charities and grandchildren and forget about any new investments for a while.

Most people wish to "minimize their maximum regret" and for most seniors, the major concern is running out of money before they die. If they encounter financial losses or major unexpected expenses, they do not have much opportunity to recover, so preservation of their money is more important than for a Second Ager. A good strategy for many to follow is to plan to keep reserves intact and curtail expenses to match income. Many planners, however, will say that spending from 5% to 8% of reserves per year (depending upon your age) is an acceptable practice, especially if the reserves are invested in growth stocks that have appreciated over the years and may not yield much current income.

These issues can be complex and many people will need outside help. The problem with that is that it is hard to find unbiased assistance. Advisors who are family members may want to maximize their eventual inheritance or may have radical ideas of what constitutes a wise investment. Banks want to generate fee income and many financial planners are most anxious to deliver a solution that generates a commission. What to do? Shop around to find an advisor/manager that you feel you can trust. Ask for references and check them out.

Managing Expenses to Match Resources

For those of modest means, extensive travel or gifts are probably not an option and a budget probably should be constructed and prioritized from the "bottom up". Some guidelines suggest that housing costs, rent or ownership costs (mortgage payments plus real estate taxes and insurance) should not exceed one-third of net monthly income. If it does, moving to a lower cost arrangement is advisable. The balance must cover food, clothing, utilities, medical expenses, transportation and entertainment. If the going gets tough, it's more pasta and less center cut, turn off the lights in the empty room, resole shoes rather than buy new ones, buy cereal in bulk rather than brand-name packages, cut out liquor, cigarettes, lottery tickets, and so on. On a positive note, a tight budget may reduce the threat of being overweight provided the food purchased is nutritious and not just inexpensive bulk. Expensive, fatty snack foods should be avoided. If an unexpected emergency expenditure is necessary, pay for it out of reserves, then plan to replace the reserves within a year at most to be ready for the next unpleasant surprise should it occur.

How big should reserves be? A suggestion is to have enough to cover the sum of the biggest unplanned, uninsured medical or dental expense plus unexpected car or home repair over the next year. Figure an amount—say $5,000. Whenever you have to dip into reserves, curtail other expenses to get back to the $5,000 within a year. This way, you'll never have to borrow money, an action unemployed seniors should try very hard to avoid. The reserves should be invested in a ready-access money-market account or equivalent that pays interest. Some seniors arrange a "reverse mortgage" using up the equity they have in their home to meet expenses. While this is low-cost borrowing that may never have to be repaid, it can result in loss of the home while it is still needed.

For those who are better off financially, there are some similarities and some differences. Housing costs may be under the one-third of income, and food plus utilities may be only a small part of the budget. There may be enough money to plan travel, gifts and various luxuries with only rarely touching reserves. Typically, in better-off families, reserves are more than enough to take care of unforeseen medical and repair bills. There may be enough money to consider the range of investments of the reserves mentioned below if they are not already in place.

Credit Cards for seniors are both a convenience and a dangerous temptation. Credit Cards enable one to avoid carrying around large amounts of cash and enable deferral of payment to a convenient time. Some cards even offer premiums like airline miles. On the other hand, there is the temptation to overspend because the pain of repayment is delayed. But credit card balances are loans at interest, usually at a very high rate. Everything winds up costing more unless balances are paid off within 30 days. Many personal bankruptcies are precipitated by excessive use of credit cards. Seniors should avoid falling into the trap of easy credit.

Investment Management

Many investment managers speak of "asset allocation". They usually are referring to: (1) the portion of reserves invested in low-risk, fixed-income investment vehicles like bonds and money market accounts, and (2) the portion of reserves invested in common stocks. One simple, often-mentioned idea is that the percentage of one's assets in fixed-income investments should equal one's age. That is, if you are 75 years old, you should have 75% of your assets safely in bonds and money market accounts and 25% at risk in stocks.

Many older investors are less risk-averse than the "age-rule" suggests and elect to have a larger portion of their holdings in stocks. They accept the added risk because they expect that stocks will increase in value in the years ahead which fixed-income investments will not do. However, if one is in failing health, it might be wise to be sure about the safety of one's assets in case the market should drop while one is incapacitated and may need cash to pay bills. Also, if one thinks that the market is overvalued and about to crash, then one might want to exercise caution by increasing the portion of one's portfolio in safer investments like bonds or money market.

To express it another way, one could say that there are two reasons for holding fixed-income, fixed-value investments like money market accounts. They are: (1) to provide a reserve for large expenditures either planned or unexpected and (2) to have a safe haven for money if the stock market seems overpriced and one wants to have cash available to take advantage of expected future buying opportunities. Brokerage houses will often publish their current recommended asset allocation. For example, they might recommend something like 20% in bonds and cash equivalents and 80% in stocks when the economic outlook is good, or perhaps 70% in bonds and cash and 30% in stocks when a general business downturn is imminent or underway.

Many people do not want to bother with this type of nervous concern and are happy to delegate the decision responsibility to a bank or investment advisor. Of course, an institution will charge a fee for this service. Often it is as much as 1% per year of the value of the account. For those with investable assets of less than $150,000, the best practice might be to invest in a "balanced" mutual fund or funds where the fund manager decides both the asset allocation and the selection of bonds and stocks. Usually the stocks selected by the fund manager are of well-established, large companies. Fidelity Puritan Fund and T. Rowe Price Equity Income Fund are examples of balanced mutual funds.

A step up in sophistication is to invest money in two ways—a percentage (say 40%) in a money market fund and the balance in a mutual fund that follows the market in general, also known as an "index" fund. Examples are the Dreyfus Money Market Fund and the Vanguard 500 Index Fund. If one wants to be somewhat more venturesome for the sake of improved chances of capital appreciation, one can direct a portion of one's investment dollars to more aggressive funds like Janus Olympus or Kaufmann Funds which are two that have had good records recently. The above examples are exactly that—examples; not recommendations. There are hundreds of mutual fund alternatives. Some have excellent records of past performance. While good past performance is a favorable sign, it is no guarantee of future performance. Some funds do well in one year, but not the next. Some have done well in a rising market only to decline badly in a falling market. It is a good idea to compare performance records before investing and to continue to make comparisons.

It may be wise to choose "no-load" funds, that is, funds where there are no purchase or exit commissions. Some funds charge a "front-end" load or salesman's commission of as much as 8%. Others levy a "back load" when redeemed. According to performance statistics, load funds do not perform any better than no-load funds. Their only advantage is that the salesman may provide helpful advice. Most "no load" funds can be purchased or redeemed by mail.

Information on the funds mentioned may be obtained by calling the following 800 numbers: Dreyfus 373-9387, Fidelity 546-8888; Janus 525-8983; Kaufmann 237-0132; T. Rowe Price 638-5660; Vanguard 662-7447. You may also wish to read the leading publication that rates mutual funds and is an excellent reference for mutual fund selection, Morningstar Fund Investor. It is issued monthly. Copies may be found in many major libraries. Also, the Friday issue of The Wall Street Journal currently lists all major mutual funds and their past performance ranking.

As mentioned above, some investors may want to strategize a bit, being heavily into a money market account if one believes the market is "too high" and more into something like the Janus Olympus fund if the market is perceived to be "near a bottom". It should be noted that very few people, however, are consistently good at identifying market tops and bottoms.

If one's investable funds are greater than about $200,000, one is probably better off buying individual stocks rather than mutual funds, provided the stocks are good choices. This is also roughly the minimum level at which one might wish to seek the services of an investment manager.

For those with the inclination, interest and analytic skill to "do it yourself", an alternate approach involves a somewhat more complex allocation process. It views the investment portfolio as composed of five categories:

Sample Percentages

1. Money market, cash equivalents   10%

2. Stable income-producing stocks like utilities,
   preferred stocks, bonds, REITs   15%

3. Established growth stocks (see sample list below)   60%

4. Cyclical stocks
   (to be bought and sold, probably not held for long term)   10%

5. Speculations—small or startup companies
   with growth potential, options, commodities   5%

   Total   100%

Category I consists of checking accounts, savings accounts, money market accounts or short-term bond funds that can be converted to cash on short notice with no shrinkage of principal. Certificates of Deposit (CD's) would be in this category from a safety standpoint, but they usually entail a penalty for early withdrawal. As suggested above, one should have enough in the way of these cash equivalents to cover large unanticipated expenses. As also mentioned above, seniors are advised to avoid incurring debts to cover unusual expenses, as it may be very difficult for them to repay loans. Some investors will also use this category as a "parking lot" for their money while awaiting advantageous investment opportunities. The percentage of one's portfolio invested in category 1, may also reflect a person's "risk profile" which will be discussed later.

Category 2 are investments made mainly for dependable income, safety and stability rather than growth. Although these investments may fluctuate in value depending on the prevailing interest rate, they are not as likely to decline very much in a bear market as other types of stocks. Utility stocks are in this category as are preferred stocks. REIT's (real estate investment trusts) would also be in category 2. Longer-term bonds of corporations, the Federal government and municipalities are in this group as would be any long-term bond mutual funds. Bond funds make sense for all but fairly large portfolios (more than $500,000) because bonds usually are in $25,000 denominations and it takes a fair amount of capital to have diversification in terms of due-date and issue. Tax-free municipal bonds yield less than taxable interest bonds but are attractive to anyone in a tax bracket of more than roughly 30%.

Category 3 includes the stocks of large, well-established companies with a strong record of growth, financial stability and good management. As of 1999, the list might include companies like General Electric, IBM, Disney, Merck, Gillette, Proctor & Gamble, AT&T, American Home Products, Pfizer, Bristol-Myers-Squibb, Johnson & Johnson, Exxon, Mobil, Chevron, Wal-Mart, American Express, Citigroup, Chase Manhattan Bank and perhaps Coca-Cola. (The list might be different in the future.) Stocks like these should be "core" holdings for dependable long-term growth.

Category 4 companies tend to be cyclical, moving up and down with the business cycle. Companies in this category today would include Boeing, General Motors, Ford, Daimler-Chrysler, International Paper, Georgia-Pacific, USX, Alcoa, Phelps-Dodge and Newmont Mining. If so inclined, one tries to buy these stocks when they seem low in the hope of selling later at a higher price. This is a risky game that is not a suitable endeavor for many people because there's a high probability of one's timing being wrong.

Category 5 stocks are those of newer companies whose products are novel and whose profitability has not been tested over a long period of time. Investments in category 5 stocks can be most rewarding if one chooses a Microsoft, Cisco, Intel, AOL, Amgen or Paychex in the early stages. The fortunes of these companies tend to be volatile and the stocks should not be purchased for those that do not understand or can't accept the associated risks.

Other speculative investments that could be included in category 5 are "Put and Call" options and commodity futures. These are highly speculative instruments in which most chance-takers lose money. They are probably not suitable for most seniors except for those with ample resources and who have a penchant for long odds and quick results, i.e. gamblers.

The percentage that one invests in each category depends on one's "time horizon", "risk profile" and ability to go a long time with investments "under water" without suffering personally. If one has ample wealth, a significant investment in promising but unproven companies may be warranted. After all, that's the essence of entrepreneurial ventures in a free economy.

If one can forego current income and would like to have a long-term gain potential, a large percentage of funds allocated to investments in Category 3 (i.e. growth stocks) is warranted. The allocation percentage depends on one's age and anticipated need for cash in the near future. If one anticipates needing cash in the next year or so, new investments in Category 3 are not advisable. Often the percentage in Category 3 "grows by itself" because of stock appreciation in value and the percentage in Category 3 grows accordingly. Disturbing this allocation, i.e. selling appreciated stock, would entail a capital gains tax liability and it may be better not to sell if only to reduce the Category 3 allocation.

If one counts on the income from investments for living expenses, travel or cash gifts, a larger allocation to income-producing investments (categories 1 & 2) is suggested. However, occasionally "sugaring off" (selling at a profit) gains in Categories 3, 4 and 5 is a way to finance special personal expenditures.

Let us look at the situation of Tom who is 70 years old and has a retirement annuity plus his Social Security of $60,000 per year. He has an investment portfolio of about $1 million. He has invested it as follows:

```
                                 XXXX
                                 XXXX
                     XX          XXXX
                     XX          XXXX
            XX       XX          XXXX      X
            XX       XX          XXXX      XX       X
Category    1        2           3         4        5
            10%      20%         60%       7.5%     2.5%
            Cash     Income      Growth    Cyclical Spec
```

This portfolio provides Tom with an additional $30,000 per year in income which adds to his financial comfort paying for some nice trips, added charitable giving and a new car every 5 years. If his Category 4 and 5 speculations pay off as he hopes, he can capture an average of another $20,000 or so per year.

Sally is different. She is a widow and her husband's survivor's pension plus Social Security amounts to $25,000 per year. She would find it hard to squeak by on that given her accustomed life style. Fortunately, she was the beneficiary of her husband's $300,000 in life insurance. She has invested that as follows:

```
                     XXXX
                     XXXX
            XXXX     XXXX
            XXXX     XXXX      XXXX
            XXXX     XXXX      XXXX
Category    1        2         3         4        5
            30%      50%       20%       0%       0%
            Cash     Income    Growth    Cyclical Spec
```

The income from these investments provide her with an extra $12,000 per year and that amount should increase a little each year and help keep up with inflation. This extra money makes the difference between being tight and being simply cautious in her financial life.

Over the long term, stocks in good companies have been excellent investments yielding better than 10% per year on average, but there are ups and downs. The stock market rose about 600% in the 17 years from 1949 to 1966. In the next 16 years, it fluctuated up and down and did not pass the 1966 high until 1983. Since that time, the market has gone up more than 900%. In between, there have been some unnerving downdrafts and more can be expected in the future. As the old saying goes, "If you can't stand the heat, stay out of the kitchen".

How does spirituality impact one's asset management? It can be said that much depends on the investor's motivation. If (s)he is using his/her money as a way to control other people or if the company in which one is investing is exploiting or victimizing customers, employees, the country or community, there isn't much spiritual merit. On the other hand, if an investor is trying to make sure that his money will last as long as he does in the face of inflation threats and trying never to be a financial burden to others, this motive has to be considered an act of thoughtfulness. In addition, if he is actively trying to improve life for his heirs or help to pay for grandchildren's' education, that's a noble objective, too. He might also be trying to develop the wherewithal to make significant gifts to his favorite school, church, hospital or other charity. Investing is all the more uplifting if money is directed toward companies that are creating products to benefit mankind and are considerate of employees, community and the environment. It does seem that these are the very companies that have been the best investments. Justice prevails.

Although the recently published book, *God is My Broker*, is largely a spoof, it does include a few words of wisdom. One rule is that "If God phones, take the call". That is to say that in selecting stocks in which to invest, good ideas sometimes come more or less out of the blue—some innovation you may have seen or read about or a product or service you see doing well. Peter Lynch, the legendary stock picker, believes in this approach. In any event, investment ideas should always be supported by research and analysis before one makes the plunge. Most major libraries have subscriptions to Standard & Poor and Value

Line investment reports, both of which are considered top information sources for stock selection.

What is a stock worth? An accepted theory is that a stock is worth the
sum of all future earnings discounted at the prevailing rate of interest.
The calculation process goes like this—make a forecast of the
company's earnings per share next year and multiply that by 1.00 minus
the current interest rate. If the current prime interest rate is 7%, the
multiplier is .93. Next, add the forecast earnings for the year after that
multiplied by .93 times .93 or .86; the year after that by .86 times .93
or .8, and so forth. Continue for a number of years ahead until the
multiplier gets quite small (roughly 10 or 15 years). Of course a forecast of a company's future earning requires considerable guesswork.
That's where extra knowledge of products and markets helps. Add it
all up and that gives the theoretical value of the stock per share.

Without going through the mathematics, it turns out that two factors
are very important: (1) the prevailing rate of interest and (2) the earnings growth rate of the company. If a company is growing steadily at a
good rate, the stock can be worth a lot in relation to current earnings,
commonly referred to at the P/E (price/earnings ratio). P is the current
market price per share. E is last year's earnings per share. If the stock
is not growing, a low P/E is appropriate (8 or so). Stocks of companies
whose earnings are in a strong uptrend (significantly higher than
current interest rates) can command PE's of 40 or more. A PE of 12
to 18 is fairly typical. A change in interest rates can affect the whole
market. A rise in interest rates tends to make stocks go down; a decline
tends to make stocks rise. Interest rates tend to be 4% plus the rate of
inflation, so inflation is generally bad for the market even though, in the
long run, company earnings should rise to reflect inflation. Also, expectations figure in. If it looks like earnings for a company will be better
than previously expected, the stock will probably rise.

It would be misleading to imply that this vast and important topic can
be summarized in a few paragraphs. In fact, a lifetime of study is
hardly enough and no one knows all the answers. How to get a handle
on the subject? Reading The Wall Street Journal or Investors Business
Daily every day and Standard & Poor's Outlook weekly is a good start.
It is interesting to note that many Wall Street titans like Cornelius

Vanderbilt, Bernard Baruch and today's Warren Buffet hit their stride after age 60.

Taking Distribution of Your 401(k) or IRA

One of the happy duties of fortunate retirees is receiving the fruits of their deferred income plan, 401(k), or Individual Retirement Account. For those who were able to set aside funds tax-free during their working years, now comes the payoff. One can begin withdrawals without penalty starting at age 59.5 and withdrawals become mandatory at age 70.5. There are 3 principal distribution options and numerous variations thereof that one can choose. Just how one selects these options depends on one's objectives. One option is to maximize the amount of money left to heirs by minimizing the withdrawals. The other extreme is to take the money in a lump sum and do "income-averaging" for tax purposes and use the money (after taxes) for whatever purpose one sees fit. An in-between option is to withdraw it all in installments that enhance your quality of life but to leave enough in the account to take care of emergencies or leave the beneficiary something, but less than the maximum.

Almost all distributions are subject to current income tax rates and, if one dies before all the money is withdrawn, the balance at death is subject to both income tax and inheritance tax. (An exception is the case where 401(k) investments were made and held in the stock of the employer and distributions are taken in the stock. In that situation, capital gains tax rates may apply.) Annual distributions can be increased, but they can't be reduced. If only you had a crystal ball to see the future, you'd know the optimum thing to do.

The example of an acquaintance, Kenny, may be helpful. Kenny worked for a major and prosperous company for many years and took advantage of their 401(K) plan starting in 1971 when he set aside half of each year's bonus. His salary was good, but not exceptional. By the time he retired at age 62 in 1985, his account stood at about $150,000. After retirement, he did some teaching and project work for several small companies, so he postponed 401(k) withdrawals until he was 70.5. By then, through judicious switching to and from a fixed income fund and an aggressive growth fund, the 401(k) had grown to $500,000. Kenny's two children were doing OK, so he didn't see the necessity of foregoing the things he wanted in order to boost their fortunes. If his wife outlived him, she would get a portion of his pension and Social Security plus she had some income of her own. In view of all that, and not wanting to die with a large balance in the 401(k) account at an advanced age, Kenny opted to withdraw $50,000 per year figuring that he would exhaust the account by about age 86. He would use the $50K (less taxes) to pay for an occasional new car and interesting travels, be a generous Santa Claus for his grand-children and have some money left over for his favorite charities or investments.

Kenny could have minimized his current taxes by withdrawing only the annual minimum which would be the value of the account divided by the combined life expectancy in years of Kenny and his wife. His wife was 2 years younger and their combined life expectancy (one or the other) was 22 years, so the minimum withdrawal was $22,700. Kenny had been increasing the value of his 401(k) more than 10% per year though smart switching of investments in the fund. He figured that if his fund performance continued that well and he withdrew only the minimum amount each year, the account would continue to grow with a big "bubble" at the end when he was too old to enjoy it and the taxes would be huge. Kenny decided to take more than the minimum.

Charitable Gift Annuities

Many seniors have had good fortune with their investments. If they have held stocks like General Electric, Coca-Cola, Merck or Proctor & Gamble for a dozen or more years, the present values are substantially more than their cost. However, these stocks are not yielding much in the way of dividends (often less than 1%) in relation to current stock prices. A person could sell the stocks and invest the proceeds in bonds that might yield 6%, but (s)he would have to pay a capital gains tax and it would take a number of years to break even.

A way for seniors with paper gains to "have their financial cake and eat it, too" is through a Charitable Gift Annuity (CGA). CGA's can be arranged by most private colleges, many churches and a host of chari-table institutions like the Nature Conservancy, Red Cross or the Salvation Army. One makes a gift of appreciated stock to the chosen charity with the understanding that the charity may sell the stock and invest the proceeds in a trust fund that yields much more than the donated stock. This income is paid to the donor for as long as (s)he lives. In addition, the donor receives a charitable gift tax deduction equal to a percentage of the value of the donated stock, depending upon the donor's age.

The benefits to the donor are the satisfaction that the gift provides resources to the chosen charity plus a tax deduction and an increase in income to the donor. Along with this is the spiritual boost that one gets from making a major gift during one's lifetime. Charitable gifts of this kind need not adversely affect heirs. If that is a concern, some or all of the increased income from the CGA can be used to purchase life insurance on the donor with heirs as beneficiaries.

Living Trusts

Wills and post-mortem trusts will be discussed later, but here are a few words about trusts as an investment management tool for the living. A person may feel unqualified to make investment decisions because they lack the education, experience, skill or interest. They may fear that they may become mentally impaired as time goes on. They may also feel pressure from other family members to make investment decisions that may be questionable. These are all reasons to set up an Irrevocable Trust in which investment management is delegated to a trustee, often a bank trust department. Another advantage of an Irrevocable Trust is that, upon the death of the person, the assets of the trust bypass probate and go directly to the beneficiaries. An alternative is a Revocable Trust, which also bypasses probate, but gives the donor the right to change or terminate the trust. A lawyer who is experienced in setting up these trusts should be consulted.

Two other types of living trusts that may be of interest to some seniors are the Grantor Retained Annuity Trust (GRAT) and the Qualified Personal Residence Trust (QPRT). The GRAT is used to designate assets to an heir and on which a gift tax is paid on the present value but the donor continues to receive the income for life or a specified period. A GRAT is a useful way to pass a farm or business to an heir. The QPRT is similar to a GRAT but pertains to the home of the donor. The donor gets life use of the residence although the ownership is passed to the heirs. Again, a lawyer who is familiar with these instruments should be consulted.

Pre-Nuptial Agreements

Third Agers contemplating remarriage often encounter conflicting interests in the disposition of financial assets upon death. These arise because an individual who has assets acquired in a previous marriage may feel an obligation to the children from that marriage and may not consider it appropriate to fully share these assets with a new partner. People can hold strong convictions on these matters and the issue has the potential of upsetting a new relationship. However, it is far better to resolve these matters before rather than after a new marriage. As unromantic as it may seem, it is advisable for the couple to explore these matters fully with a lawyer and try to reach an agreement. These agreements may extend to division and application of income and use of property as well as assets. Marriage may result in the loss of income for one or both members of the couple. If the financial penalty of marriage is severe enough, the couple may decide against marriage and enjoy a "relationship". Even then, a formal agreement may be designed to address financial and property matters of mutual concern.

Risk Management for Seniors

Many seniors worry a lot about the potentially adverse things that could befall them late in life over which they have little or no control. Severe physical and mental health problems, auto and other accidents, general frailty, the process of dying, family disasters, property damage and theft, a crashing stock market and runaway inflation are common concerns.

It is important to face these issues squarely. Denial about potential problems, particularly things like driving or impending disability, may postpone precautionary decisions or measures beyond the time when remedial steps can be taken. For example, long term health care insurance becomes very expensive after age 70 and is unobtainable if a serious health condition develops.

Regarding long-term health care insurance, it has been said that 4 out of 5 people are better off being self-insured, that is, designating enough personal assets to cover the cost of long term health care. Most people will die at home, with their children, in the hospital or after a short stay in a hospice or nursing home. Less than 20% will be in a nursing home for an extended period of time, that is, a number of years. (However, a typical stay for an Alzheimer's patient is 4 to 8 years.) If a person has depleted his or her assets, Medicaid will cover the cost of long-term care. But then, many nursing homes are refusing Medicaid patients or those who have insufficient assets to cover a long stay because they cannot provide quality service profitably for the reimbursement allowed. Facilities that will accept Medicaid patients are often crowded and understaffed. In any event, unless one has substantial assets to pledge, long term health insurance is a good idea to enhance admission prospects to a preferred facility. Even if one has sufficient assets, one may want this insurance to dispel anxieties by family and to be worry-free in this regard during the well years. Also, with long-term health care insurance, one can be more aggressive in investments and less conservative in expenditure. Finally, the composure that comes with reduced worry may boost one's outlook on life's remainder.

If one has a desire to travel, the more strenuous or adventurous trips should be taken when one is able rather than waiting because one never knows what next year will bring. Even challenges like negotiating the Paris Metro may become difficult if arthritis limits stair climbing. Without doubt, each passing year decreases the probability that some types of travels can be taken without a mishap. Call it a "shrinking window of opportunity". In any event, everyone over age 65 should consider buying trip-cancellation insurance for major trips that have non-refundable payments. If traveling with a spouse, one should get the type of insurance contract that covers both even if only one cannot make the trip. Most insurance companies will require a doctor's statement, so one should be in contact with his or her doctor regarding any condition that would prevent the trip. Also, even though most seniors have medical (Medicare) insurance, which should cover medical service abroad, it may be wise to get extra coverage for foreign trips because Medicare may require verification that may be difficult to obtain. Other types of concerns, especially accidents and thefts, may be addressed by realistic planning and by taking precautions. Some wit once said, "Most accidents happen in the home, so play it safe, don't go home". Similarly, most auto accidents happen within 5 miles of home. Lapses in concentration, loss of balance, denial regarding diminishing physical capability or failing memory can be the cause of accidents for the elderly. Activities that used to be simple, like replacing the light bulb in a ceiling fixture, now may require help. Bathrooms with wet surfaces represent a disaster waiting to happen, so grab bars should be installed within easy reach and tub mats should be in place. Use of upper shelves of cupboards and closets that need a stepladder for access should be used only to store seldom-used items. Special tools are available to extend the reach and grasp. Containers that weigh more than 10 pounds when full should be avoided. Heavy suitcases are a common cause of back injury. Always lift straight up using legs rather than straining back. Do not lift with a jerk; use a steady force. A cane or walking stick for support and balance should be used when walking over uneven ground. Check the soles of shoes for wear that would make them slippery. Also, select shoes with good traction as well as support—let style be secondary to safety.

In today's society, an automobile has become a near-necessity, so restricting or giving up driving can be more than just an inconvenience, it can be demoralizing. Nevertheless, a time may come when a person must come to grips with the problem of declining capability and the associated dangers. Some states require requalifying driving tests for persons over 70. Even if one passes, there are some limitations that can develop that call for special judgements. Reaction times that are slower, eyesight that has deteriorated and lapses in concentration are deficiencies that come with age. To compensate, seniors should avoid driving after dark, particularly in unfamiliar places; avoid rush hour traffic; avoid freeways that have complicated or frequent merges or crossovers. If you never pass anyone, you are probably the slowest one on the road and therefore a possible obstacle to other drivers. Take the slow lane or road where you are less likely to bother others. Slow drivers seeing a line-up behind should pull off the road to let the others pass. Drive defensively. Seniors should take the 55 ALIVE course offered by AARP, AAA and other organizations to review and correct bad driving habits. Beware of other people in slow-moving cars and be prepared for irrational acts like left turns with right signal blinking. Try not to be one of them. If a spouse or friend collides frequently with parked cars, it's time to hang up the car keys for good. They must be told the bad news. All of these sad eventualities are better tolerated if one is spiritually mindful of the needs of others. Finally, in view of the fact that those over 70 tend to get into more accidents than 50-year-olds, it is a good idea for seniors to drive a car that provides safety in the event of a collision. Air bags and fastened seat belts are a good idea. Also, a heavier car is a safer car even though they may cost more to buy and operate.

Another risk that seniors face is the chance of being mugged or being a purse-snatching victim. Hoodlums perceive the elderly as easy targets. Rule number one is stay out of hoodlum neighborhoods, especially after dark. Unfortunately, hoodlum neighborhoods seem to be spreading, so it may not always be possible to stay away. The next best approach is to have a well-attached cellular phone in plain view to let the thug know you are only seconds from dialing 911. (A cell phone can be even more effective than a gun in warding off attackers.) An expendable decoy wallet or purse containing a few dollars but no credit cards or valuable documents should be handed over willingly to a thief. It's better to lose a few dollars than your life. Consider carrying a loud whistle and maybe a mace squirter, where legal, but be careful, use of these may provoke a thug into violent action. A check with local police may offer additional ideas for self-protection. A cellular phone is also useful in case of car breakdowns on the highway, physical distress away from home, or even a fall inside the home away from the regular phone. Similarly, cordless phones in the home are useful to take into the bathroom or garage in case of an emergency.

In any event, it is practical and realistic to think through every situation regarding what could go wrong and try to take some precaution. However, one must reach a balance, especially with regard to travel. If you worry too much about what could go wrong, you might become a hermit. For the sake of making the most of the shrinking window of opportunity for adventure, self-esteem and spiritual uplift, one simply has to accept some risk and go forth.

Summarizing the thoughts in this chapter, money and risks are key issues for seniors. It has often been said that money doesn't buy happiness. A joking line in *God is My Broker* says that money doesn't buy happiness until you spend it. It is not necessary to have great wealth to be happy, but sufficient money does provide resources for options, choices, safety and comfort. Often this equates with happiness. Even if it is too late in life for one to enhance his or her finances, we can send an important message to the anti-establishment flower children of the 1960's and their followers. For most seniors, an enjoyable, fulfilling and spiritually uplifted Third Age is predicated on having enough money. Young idealists are foolish to think otherwise.

> "If I had my life to live over,
> I would take more chances.
> I would take more trips.
> I would climb more mountains and swim more rivers.
> Perhaps I would have more actual troubles,
> but I'd have fewer imaginary ones.
> I would pick more daisies."
>
> —Nadine Stair at age 85.

V

Physical, Mental and Emotional Wellness Enjoying A Longer and Healthier Third Age Of Life

Ideas for: Promoting Mental Wellness and Avoiding Depression; Coping with Alzheimer's Disease; Improving Relations with Spouse and Others; Self-Empowerment. Understanding: Mind/Body Interactions and the "Three-Legged Stool" of Health Care—Medication, Treatment and Self-Help. Information regarding: Healthy Eating Habits—Nutrition, Diet, and Weight Control; Longer and Better Life through Exercise and Physical Activity; Sexual Fulfillment for Seniors.

The Third Age of life can be threatening. Often the morale of seniors is undermined by the loss of the career they left behind when they retired. They may miss the stimulus of their working days. Perhaps younger people took over toward the end and eased them aside in their organizations. While that's a normal course of events, it may be difficult to accept and resentment, anxiety, loss of self-esteem and depression may result. Add to that declining physical ability, perhaps tentative finances, loss of friends and an unsympathetic spouse with his or her own problems and life in retirement can seem dreary. In spite of all this, we should know that the Third Age can be the best age of all. These are years that can be wonderfully fulfilling and in which seniors can grow spiritually. But, to be spiritually uplifted and face each day with enthusiasm, it helps to feel good physically and mentally. This chapter offers a number of suggestions to enhance good feelings about oneself.

Mental Wellness and Avoiding Depression

Depression is common among seniors, but depression is readily treatable and anyone who notices the symptoms listed below or recognizes them in one's spouse or partner, should seek help from their family physician (PCP) or mental health professional. Any five or more of the following symptoms that persist for more than two weeks are cause for action.

* Persistent sad, anxious or "empty" mood or severe loneliness.
* Sleeping too little or too much.
* Unintended changes in weight or appetite.
* Diminished interest or pleasure in most or all activities.
* Extended time looking vacantly into space or at a blank wall.
* Persistent physical symptoms, like diarrhea or headaches that don't respond to treatment.
* Difficulty concentrating, remembering or making decisions.
* Frequent fatigue or loss of energy.
* Feeling unliked, guilty, hopeless, helpless or worthless.
* Frequent excessive alcohol consumption.
* Recurrent thoughts of suicide.
* Behavioral changes like apathy, explosive anger, and constant criticism of others or unfounded suspicion.

Persistent and severe depression is an illness that is often caused by a chemical imbalance in the brain of the neurotransmitter, seritonin.

The onset of depression may be triggered by a traumatic experience like the loss of a spouse, a move or the loss of stimulation resulting from retirement, but often it is for no apparent reason at all. Depression cannot be detected by pulse or fever or any other measurable symptom. It is diagnosed by answers to a number of questions, many of which are suggested by the list above. If your doctor believes it will help, he is likely to prescribe one of several medications that have helped millions of people cope with stress, anxiety and depression. The current list includes Prozac. Zoloft, Paxil, Effexor, Bupropion, BuSpar and Serzone. It is often appropriate to combine medication with therapy to help develop a "new and improved" view of life. This might start by formulating one's "vision" of an ideal life within one's financial and physical limitations. The next step would be to develop a set of initiatives to achieve the vision. (Go back to Chapter III for ideas.) One should not overlook the importance of spiritual renewal as an aid to constructing a more positive view of life. Although some people still may avoid professional help for depression because of the stigma sometimes associated with mental illness, widespread publicity has made this a lesser problem. It is pointless to suffer due to denial when capable and effective help is readily available.

Alzheimer's Disease and Coping with it.

Neurologist and lecturer, Dr. Randolph Schiffer tells us that the most dreaded illness for seniors today is Alzheimer's Disease. It used to be that cancer was the most dreaded, but great advances in cancer treatment have ameliorated that fear. Alzheimer's is so troubling because it often involves a total loss of everything a person values—humor, intelligence, mobility, dignity and, perhaps most of all, their spirituality. It's usually of long duration and takes a terrible toll on caregivers and often finances. Some view it as a fate worse than death.

Dr. Schiffer indicates that there is growing evidence that there is a genetic link or predisposition to Alzheimer's and that it does not seem to be caused by diet or virus or anything else in the environment, except possibly it is triggered by stress. He does not subscribe to the notion that aluminum cooking utensils are a cause, contrary to some speculation. Fortunately, it appears that there are several things a person can do to delay the onset and there are new medications

(Aricept) that may also delay or mitigate the effects. A disease delayed long enough is almost the equivalent of a cure. So there's hope.

Studies show that Alzheimer's is, on the average, a 12-year illness. Currently, there are no lab tests that lead to a diagnosis. Even if there were, they would be pointless because there is no cure. However, there are tests that measure a patient's ability in logic, visual and motor skills as well as manifestations of significant memory and behavioral changes. (Only an autopsy after death can confirm the disease.) Alzheimer's disease typically begins with cognitive deterioration. Characteristics are: loss of memory (can't remember children's' names or the way home from nearby places), loss of arithmetic skills (difficulty making change or maintaining checkbook), loss of abstract skills (can't read a map or clock), loss of small muscle skills (difficulty dressing oneself or non-arthritic deteriorating handwriting) and perception skills (failing to see stop signs or red lights). If these symptoms become quite apparent, a doctor should be consulted. Forgetting where one left one's car keys is not a symptom of Alzheimer's, but forgetting what the keys are for is a sign of trouble.

Typically, these losses progress for about 4 years before skills are so diminished that a person cannot care for oneself. Then it is time for family members to consider other options for the person such as day care, home care or nursing home. Dr. Schiffer says to expect about 8 years before brain damage eventually affects respiration and the heart fatally. Of course, the exact duration will vary from one person to another.

There is an unproven belief by many experts that cholesterol deposits affect the brain as well as arteries and that cholesterol-lowering medications like Mevacor, Zocor and Prevachol help to delay the onset or progress of Alzheimer's. Many doctors suggest that an aspirin every day or two may be beneficial. Brain exercises like crossword puzzles, computer work or card games also seem to help to keep the mind in shape and enhance memory retrieval and reasoning.

As soon as any dementia symptoms are recognized, it is important that one's lawyer is notified so that key decisions such as will making and the making of living wills, health proxies, trusts, and powers of attorney may be executed. Better yet, these things will have been settled before the onset of any loss of mental prowess and while the person is regarded as competent so that important decisions will not be challenged later. Once the disease takes hold, the patient may exhibit difficulty in making decisions and anger combined with paranoia may develop. Alzheimer's patients rarely commit suicide, but they may become hostile and resentful. The disease is probably hardest on the caregivers, and they should reserve time and money for themselves without guilt. The only spiritual benefit that may derive from a loved one's Alzheimer's may come from the kindness, tolerance, and sacrifice and love that the caregiver musters. In this regard it may help to focus on the person's "good years".

Individuals with Alzheimer's symptoms should give up driving as soon as symptoms become apparent. Hopefully (s)he will do this willingly. If not, the family or the attending physician should check state laws on the subject and perhaps notify the state Bureau of Motor Vehicles. In some states, this can be done anonymously, in which case, the DMV can demand a driving exam, which, if not passed, will result in a revocation of license. Although this action may seem intrusive, getting the impaired driver off the road is in everybody's interest. The disabled person may still be able to participate in the driving process by pumping gas and cleaning the windshield.

If an Alzheimer's patient has a spouse who is still lively, sociable and perhaps even adventurous, questions of fidelity arise. Should the healthy spouse date or travel with a person of the opposite sex? Should there be a divorce, perhaps for financial reasons? These are difficult questions about which the healthy spouse might seek advice from his or her lawyer or clergy-person and follow the dictates of their own conscience. Whatever the decision, others should withhold judgement.

On an optimistic note, many pharmaceutical laboratories have attached a high priority to work on medications that will postpone or suppress Alzheimer's symptoms. As of this writing, Aricept is a new prescription medication that seems to help mild to moderate dementia of the Alzheimer's type. Hopefully more good news will be forthcoming in the near future.

Improving Relations with Spouse and Others

When one or both members of a couple retire, they are bound to spend a lot more time with each other. This can be a joyous time or a test of "for better or worse". Any incompatibilities that existed before retirement are greatly magnified simply through increased exposure after retirement. According to psychologist and lecturer, Dr. C. Marrett Lacey, the ideal marriage includes mutual commitment, intimacy, passion, shared values and good communication. When any part of this mix is missing, the potential for deterioration of the relationship arises. That's unfortunate because in the Third Age a husband and wife usually need each other and, if they can't get along harmoniously, the years ahead can be painful rather than enjoyable.

Many long-time marriages are demonstrations of commitment. However, commitment by itself may be a rather empty relationship especially when children are out of the equation. What may have evaporated over the years are the romance of intimacy and passion and the excitement of new joint projects. Remarriages may have the romance but an untested commitment. The new spouse may have only minimal appreciation for what the life of the other person was like in the early years and the challenges that were met back then. For long-term marriages that have become dull or troubled, sincere attempts to regenerate the old excitement can be successful. An effort to enhance spirituality has provided uplift to rejuvenate some marriages. Marriage Encounter groups organized through many churches pursue this approach. More information may be obtained from International Marriage Encounter, 955 Lake Drive, St. Paul, MN 55120 or phone 1-800-MARRIAGE.

Shared values are similar viewpoints regarding interests like travel, hobbies, or sports; allocation of time and money; care-giving and time spent with children and grandchildren; politics or religion. Even in the best of marriages, it is too much to expect that the values will be precisely alike, but they should be reasonably close for harmony. At age 60 or 70 or so, one cannot expect another person to change very much. Areas of discord may have to be overlooked, tolerated or "worked around", at least up to some point. To help in this process, Dr. Lacey recommends that troubled couples compose separate lists of things they like about each other and their shared values. The key to rekindling romance may be in focusing on the items of mutual appreciation. That may require a conscious effort and the planning of activities of joint interest. Try to generate pleasant surprises.

If the list of shared interests or values is rather short, conflict and control issues may develop in the retirement years. The following is a quote from Dr. Lacey's work. "This (Third Age) is often a time when couples recognize that many individual interests have changed and they need to reach an acceptance that each partner will occasionally pursue activities that do not involve the other partner. As the partnership matures without possessiveness and with trust, one may recognize that with aging, time may be shorter. It is therefore important for a spouse to accept and even encourage the partner to pursue his/her own dream. A spouse needs to recognize that pursuit of separate interests, travel, sports and perhaps some life style changes will not threaten the relationship. Also, everyone should have a location that is his or her private domain. A place in the home, an office, a camp in the woods or a boat or RV. The antithesis of this is the situation where one partner makes it apparent that he/she has a need to control the life of the other partner. Often one person gives in to the other to avoid the harassment, resents the control and often is intimidated. This may result in a divisive atmosphere instead of an environment where both partners believe they are in control of their own lives. This is an example of the need for self-empowerment to have a healthy environment. If this is too difficult to achieve, then one or both partners should consider counseling with a professional. Visits to a professional and state-licensed therapist or social worker, in order to be successful, must be continuous for a period of time and involve honesty on the part of the client. There should be limited complaining and playing helpless or victimized. A complaining client that wants a therapist who puts a "band aid" on the hurt is not a long-term solution. The more valued therapist will help guide the client and enable the client to develop his/her own awareness. Part of the process of developing an awareness of one's self may involve some emotional discomfort. This is understandable since habits, attitudes and behaviors develop over many years. Therefore one cannot expect immediate happiness or answers to all the problems in just a few sessions." Even couples who have been married a long time, may have to make some major adjustments in their relationships in retirement.

Self-Empowerment

Self-empowerment is the ability to be oneself and not be manipulated by those who might want to control you or want you to accept substandard service or product. The controllers might be spouse, children or others with influence. Back in one's working days one may have had to accept a controlling boss or move on. You were being paid to accept someone else's direction. Retirement ought to be a time to be free of that stress and be your own person.

In the Third Age, most seniors no longer have the "clout" that may have formerly accompanied leadership or key positions in established organizations. As previously mentioned, the world often takes advantage of a senior's diminished power by trying to get them to buy something they don't want or need, make decisions that are unfair to the senior or accept substandard service or goods. There is no one to crown you "King or Queen of the Hill"; you have to grab your own power. It is not necessary to be obnoxious,, but to get quality service and treatment from salespeople, civil servants, repairmen, waitresses and medical personnel, you often have to be assertive.

Although unfair, people often judge strangers by their appearance and expression. Self-presentation is important—you must look smart, act convincingly, dress well, arrive in a clean car, stand tall and speak up. Act like you are financially secure even if you have reservations. Know clearly what you want and go after it. Resist compromises. Don't apologize where no apology is due. Demand what is rightfully yours. Don't hesitate to go or write to a superior if you have been mistreated by a service person. Even if in a hospital or nursing home, one must not suffer silently. As always and everywhere, the "squeaky wheel gets the grease".

A person who is depressed from the loss of a spouse, particularly a spouse who was the more assertive one in the family, or has been left with meager finances may find it hard to be more aggressive. Assertiveness training from an organization like OASIS may be very useful.

Self-empowerment means being self-reliant and in control of one's life and does not mean being obtrusive or hostile. If a person is motivated by a sincere desire for fairness to all concerned, self-empowerment will boost self-esteem and be spiritually uplifting.

A corollary to self-empowerment is survivorship. This is a mind-set that is a determination to outlive a financial, emotional and/or physical disaster. One can imagine a bankrupt business, a severe auto accident that results in a major injury, an uninsured house fire, abandonment by a spouse and many other possibilities that could change one's life leaving one in a desperate condition. If not affected oneself, one may want to counsel a downhearted friend who may have experienced a personal loss. Fortunately, our society has some safety nets—welfare, Medicaid and numerous charitable organizations that one can fall back on. Pride may have to be overlooked. The victim needs to become highly resourceful in obtaining food, clothing and shelter. Often church clergy can provide helpful counseling. There are no cure-all suggestions. All persons are advised to organize their life so that tragedies are anticipated as well as possible and so that they don't happen without protection or a "fall back" alternative action.

Mind-Body Interactions

Deterioration of the body due to age-related ailments like arthritis, heart trouble, vision or hearing loss or other serious problems like emphysema or Parkinson's disease is very likely to have an adverse effect on the mind, maybe even precipitating severe depression. Less obvious is the effect of the mind on the body—the idea that our thoughts can influence our health. This is not a new concept. Some will say that this was the power source of Jesus' reported miracles. Mary Baker Eddy, in founding the Church of Christ, Scientist in 1879, had this as one of the guiding principles. Christian Scientists continue to believe strongly that most physical problems (with exceptions like broken bones and dentistry) can be healed by faith and prayer.

There is a growing amount of scientific evidence that stress and attitude can bring about chemical changes in the body that can affect the immune system and healing process in positive or negative ways. More than 300 scientific studies report that religious commitment is associated with better health. According to Dr. Dale Matthews of Georgetown School of Medicine, twenty years ago thoughts like this would have brought chuckles and snide remarks in medical school. By contrast, some medical schools now offer courses about the influence of the mind on healing.

Studies have been conducted that show that religious and spiritual beliefs can contribute to an improved ability to prevent or combat physical disorders like heart disease, cancer, high blood pressure, addiction or depression. Belief in a higher power is the cornerstone of the therapy of Alcoholics Anonymous. Religiously committed people are often found to recover quicker from surgery and enjoy a longer life expectancy—9 years for men, 4 for women in one Dutch Study.

The spiritual uplift that has been described herein is meant to promote optimism, hope, a sense of purpose and connection to community and family. This spirit buffers stress and offers peace and comfort in times of trouble. Familiar rituals and prayer have been known to produce salutary changes in one's pulse, blood pressure and metabolic rate.

Dr. Herbert Benson of Harvard Medical School and the Mind/Body Medical Institute is the author and/or co-author of several books on mind/body interactions: *Timeless Healing: The Power and Biology of Belief, The Relaxation Response, The Mind/Body Effect, Beyond the Relaxation Response and Your Maximum Mind*. Probably better recognized than any other current writer on the subject, Dr. Benson has studied and promoted the value of understanding the effect of the mind on the body.

The "Three-Legged Stool of Health Care"

Dr. Benson has a basic idea that is easy to grasp. He describes health care and physical wellness as a "Three-Legged Stool":

Leg 1-Medication
Leg 2-Treatment, including Surgery and diagnostics
Leg 3-SELF HELP

Medication, Leg #1, is widely (but not universally) accepted as a first step in curing a disease. Many medications have a long history of success. New drugs that have been developed in the past 50 years have produced miracles in curing, controlling or preventing many diseases that were thought to be fatal a generation ago. Additional advances keep coming along yearly. These drugs have been a major factor in improving longevity as well as physical and mental health.

It must be noted that many people, for various reasons, lack confidence in these medications and prefer "alternative" or homeopathic treatments like herbal medicines or acupuncture. Popular "food supplement" alternatives are ginko biloba, ginseng, kava, saw palmetto and St. John's wort. These are called "alternative" because they are not endorsed by the American Medical Association, which organization questions their effectiveness, purity and/or safety. Also, they are not subject to approval by the Food & Drug Administration (FDA). While almost all medications have side effects and many simply don't work for some individuals, on balance, prescription medications do much more good than harm and the best policy is to accept the advice of a professional with access to complete information. Compared to the extensive testing of ethical drugs required by the FDA, few herbs and botanical remedies have been rigorously studied for effectiveness, side effects or interactions with other substances. Also there is no standardization. They are considered technically to be food supplements rather than medications and thereby escape FDA scrutiny. Nevertheless, the increasing use of alternatives has caused many physicians within the AMA to call for definitive answers regarding the use of alternatives.

Unfortunately, many of the new prescription medications are expensive and are beyond many budgets. Medicare currently does not pay for medications and HMOs may call for large co-payments. This is a major reason some doctors recommend and why many people have chosen to use alternatives—simply because they are usually much less expensive. Also, many people avoid medications altogether because they fear that they may contaminate the body. Still others limit themselves to "natural" remedies. It should be noted that many "natural" substances are highly toxic. Without doubt, public discussion on this issue will continue in the future.

Treatment, Leg #2, includes surgery, hospital care, physical and mental therapy, organ transplants, prostheses, consultation and anesthesia as well as lab tests and diagnostics. Although the quality of treatment may vary by facility and location, undeniable and significant progress has been achieved almost everywhere in recent years. The big problem is that health care has become ever more costly for a variety of reasons mostly related to improved technology along with increased longevity. In an effort to control costs, some Managed Care plans have limited the access to some treatments and reduced allowable hospital time. Seniors are well-advised to use their influence to resist reductions in quality of care.

SELF HELP, Leg #3, covers many personal interventions, some physical, some mental. Dr. Benson is a leading thinker on this subject and his books describe a number of aspects of self help. He talks about a relaxation response, remembered wellness, faith, prayer, diet, exercise, healthy distractions and positive thinking. His books cover these subjects in much more detail than is attempted here.

Relaxation is both mental and physical and is a method to reduce stress, which affects the immune system and wellness. The relaxation method involves a conscious relaxation of the muscles by flexing them, then releasing them one at a time. Included is a deliberate control of breathing—deep inhalation followed by slow exhalation, repetitiously. It also suggests imaging of restful thoughts with closed eyes; purging the mind of anxious thoughts; and listening to restful sounds—those of mountain streams, ocean waves or soft music. Tai Chi exercises can be included. This relaxation ritual might well become a daily routine. At night before retiring is a convenient time to practice relaxation but it is not the only possibility. While waiting for a bus or plane or standing in a waiting line are other opportunities.

If one is suffering from an illness, instead of focusing on the pain or discomfort, one should try to think back to a time when one felt "very good" and what it was like. Dr. Benson refers to this as "remembered wellness". It seems to help many people. Similarly, in medication trials, it is interesting to observe that placebos are as much as 30% as effective as the medication being tested and the only explanation is a mind/body interaction.

The "Faith Factor" is the belief in something good, whether it is the God of a particular religion, another person held in high esteem, like one's doctor, or faith in the treatment one is receiving. In connection with religious faith, for sincere believers, prayer has been found to be convincingly beneficial. A person should not submit to a treatment in which they do not have faith. One's attitude and belief in the effectiveness of a procedure is known to enhance recovery.

Healthy Eating Habits

Is there any senior who doesn't realize that proper diet and nutrition are important for good health and longevity? In spite of wide publicity, an alarmingly large percentage of American people are obese or overweight and seniors are no exception. In addition to the health risk, obese people are often rejected socially and suffer from isolation. In view of the bad effects of being overweight, why do so many people have trouble controlling their eating habits?

The problem seems to be cultural. Food can be an expression of love, eating with others is sociable, food is fun, eating is "something to do". Most of all, we are barraged with food advertising and alluring packaging. Man is the only animal that eats more than his needs. Some wives express their devotion to family by preparing inviting meals with generous portions. Restaurants try to give a "good value" by loading up the plates with calories. "Lets do lunch" is often an invitation to guzzle and gorge. Perhaps the height of excess food is the gluttonous late evening "snack" on a cruise ship. While watching TV, having a bag of goodies to dip into provides oral gratification to offset the tension on the screen. Some of the most talented artists of our time are engaged to design advertisements and gorgeous packaging for high fat foods that are so tempting that when mama pushes her cart down the supermarket aisle, she often cannot pass without grabbing the beautiful delight on the shelf. If dad is the shopper, he's probably just as guilty. (Rarely are carrot or celery sticks promoted.) Even the "low fat" foods are deceptive because they often substitute sugar for fat to make the product taste good. One must read container labels carefully to know what one is getting. The neon and dazzling lights of the fast-food joints beckon the tired, the lonely and the bored as well as the hungry, and proceed to tempt them with fat-loaded taste treats. TV ads plead with children to urge their (grand)parents to buy low-nutrition treats. It seems that the less healthy the food, the more the customers return. Then there is the problem of alcohol and the infamous cocktail party—lots of calories and little or no nutrition—to say nothing of the other problems of too much alcohol. It becomes a setup for failure and loss of self–control.

How do those who are overweight deal with the problem? The answer includes education and self-discipline. Here's where spirituality and belief in something good can help. If one accepts the idea that an important goal in our Third Age is to stay healthy in order to be useful to oneself and others, then we have a strong motivation to develop and maintain healthy eating habits. For those who say grace before meals, perhaps a plea for fortitude to take small helpings and leave the table before feeling full will help.

There are two parts to healthy eating—limit the quantity of food to the right total amount and be sure that the various food groups are consumed in the right proportions for proper nutrition. Numerous books on diet and nutrition, many of which can be purchased off the shelf in drug stores and supermarkets, will provide the details, but probably the most authoritative source is the US Department of Agriculture and their various inexpensive publications. The publication, *Dietary Guidelines for Americans* is a best-seller and costs only 50 cents. It can be ordered from the Center for Nutrition Policy & Promotions, 1120 20th St. NW, Suite 200, Washington, DC 20036; phone (202) 606-8000.

There are a few textbook nutrition facts that are worth keeping in mind. A pound of body fat represents 3600 calories. Just through breathing, the heart pumping and giving off body heat, a person burns about 13 calories per pound of body weight each day. If you exercise or are physically active, especially in cold air, it goes up to 16 to 18 calories per pound of body weight. In other words, a 150-pound person who sits at a desk all day will use up about 2000 calories per day. To lose a pound of body fat, a person must burn 3600 calories more than one consumes in food. So, if the 150-pound person at the desk all day goes on a 1500 calories-per-day diet, he or she can expect to lose a pound about every 8 days or 5 pounds in about 40 days. Now, if the

150 pound person is quite active physically, hiking, gardening or painting the house, he or she will use up about 2700 calories per day. Then, if that person goes on a 1500 calories-per-day diet, he or she can expect to lose a pound about every 3 days or 5 pounds in about 15 days. Weight loss programs usually do not advise a diet of less than 1000 calories per day (1200 for men) in order to have adequate nutrition. Therefore, one has to be patient with weight loss. Ads that claim that 10 pounds can be lost in a week are misrepresentations in that they are talking about loss of water, not fat, and the weight comes right back with the next drink. Also, these "crash" programs are dangerous in that they may result in dehydration.

A way to determine if a person is overweight is through a computation of the Body Mass Index (BMI). Readers can calculate their BMI by multiplying their weight by 700 and dividing by their height in inches squared. (For example, I weigh 195 pounds and am 70 inches tall, so my BMI is 28.) A desirable BMI is between 19 and 25; 25 to 30 is overweight and over 30 suggests obesity. (I know what I need to do.) A waist-hip ratio is another way of assessing body composition. The ideal ratio is less than .8 for women and below 1.0 for men. (For example, I have a waist of 38 inches and hips of 43 inches for a ratio of .88.) People with apple-shaped bodies have large waist-to-hip ratios. It has been said that "Apples" are candidates for heart disease and "Pears", with smaller waist-to-hip ratios, are less likely to have heart trouble.

When a person is at his or her ideal weight, or at least a weight at which he or she feels good, then a maintenance diet of 13 to 18 calories per day per pound of body weight (depending on activity level) is appropriate. For a person who is content with a weight of 150 Pounds, a maintenance diet would be 1950 to 2700 calories per day. For a maintenance diet in calories for other body weights, one has to go through the arithmetic multiplying

13 (or 14 to 18 depending on activity level) by the desired body weight. As always, dieting should be done with the supervision of a qualified dietician, doctor or reputable weight loss clinic.

One really has to count calories in order to know when the allowable calories per day have been reached. Most diet books will include a calorie table. It's a good idea to become familiar with such a table, knowing especially the calorie content of one's favorite foods and customary portions.

The so-called FOOD PYRAMID, defined by the U.S. Department of Agriculture, is a device to make understandable the essentials of good nutrition. It is expressed as servings per day and is as follows:

Servings per Day	Food Groups
1	Fat, oils or sweets
2 or 3	Milk, yogurt or cheese
2 or 3	Meat, Poultry, fish, beans, eggs or nuts
2 to 4	Fruits
3 to 5	Vegetables
6 to 11	Cereal, bread, rice or pasta

This all becomes more meaningful when it is translated into a menu of foods that you like and are likely to eat. For example: a half grapefruit and a bowl of shredded wheat with 1% fat milk, no sugar, black coffee for breakfast; Greek salad and apple for lunch; roast chicken breast, baked potato (no sour cream or butter) carrots and spinach for dinner with cupcake for dessert. In addition to covering the food groups, one should also make sure that the total calories are within the dietary goals.

Calorie and nutrient tables for a long list of foods can be found in the booklets available in supermarkets. They should be studied and memorized well enough so that one can estimate the calorie content of a meal without having to refer constantly to the tables. One suggestion that has been offered to those who are trying to improve their diet is to keep a "Food Diary". This is a list of foods eaten during the day. At the end of the day, or whenever convenient, one can go through the list and add up the calories and make sure they are within guidelines and that nutrient requirements have been met.

Vitamins are natural chemical components of foods that have little or no caloric content but are necessary for good health. Different foods have very different vitamin contents. Many authorities will say that a daily menu that contains all the food groups of the Pyramid in normal quantities should take care of most vitamin requirements. Those on a diet of less than 1500 calories per day may have trouble meeting nutrient requirements and extra vitamins may be necessary for proper nutrition. Others may benefit from vitamin supplements, as indicated below. Currently, there are more than 7000 books in print dealing with nutrition and diet. Probably the most authoritative source of information, currently, is The American Dietetic Association's *Complete Food & Nutrition Guide* by Roberta Larson Duyff. The book points out that there are 13 vitamins that are currently recognized as essential for good health: A (beta carotene), B1 (thiamin), B2 (riboflavin), B3 (niacin), B5 (pantothenic acid), B6, B12, C (ascorbic acid), D, E, H and K. and folic acid. The National Academy of Science has established Recommended Dietary Allowances (RDA's), the amount of each vitamin that should be consumed daily for good health. However, these recommendations have come under question in light of recent research and there is evidence that the present RDA's are too low, especially for older persons and that vitamin intake in excess of the RDA's is beneficial.

Below is a condensed list of vitamins and their present RDA's, their sources and benefits. (It should be emphasized that this information is subject to change and is presented mainly as a "benchmark" against future recommendations.)

Vitamin	RDA	Source	Benefits
A (beta carotene)	1000 IU	Dairy products, green vegetables	Vision, tissue Immune system
B1 (thiamin)	1.5 mg	Cereals, fish lean meat	Heart, growth,energy
B2 (riboflavin)	1.7 mg	Cereals, dairy products, lean meat	Tissue repair, antibodies
B3 (niacin)	18 mg	Cereals, lean meat	Nervous system, skin
B5 (pantothenic acid)	7mg	Vegetables	Energy, immune system

B6 (pyradoxine)	2 mg	Vegetables	Red blood cells
B12 (cyanocobalamine)	3 mg	Milk, fish, lean meat	Red blood cells
C (ascorbic acid)	60 mg	Citrus fruits	Immune system, Anti-oxidant, blood
D	400 IU	Sunshine, fish, milk	Bones, teeth
E	30 IU	Wheat germ	Anti-oxidant, HDL, tissue repair
H (biotin)	200 mg	Eggs, leafy Vegetables	Metabolism
K (menadione)	Not established	Leafy green vegetables	Blood clotting
Folic acid	400 mg	Leafy vegetables	Intestinal tract

The Produce Marketing Association publishes tables of the vitamin content of a large number of foods. They point out, however, that the vitamin content of foods can vary and depends on the composition of the soil, water, fertilizer and growing conditions and other factors at the source. The complexity involved makes it almost impossible for people to know their exact vitamin intake from the food they eat. The National Academy of Science has said that large segments of the population should take vitamin supplements, even people who try to eat a well-balanced diet. Seniors in particular, because of possible denture problems and loss of smell or taste and demands of the immune system, may not be getting all the nutrients that they should. For this reason, many authorities recommended that seniors, especially, take a vitamin supplement. Furthermore, various studies indicate that there may be value in taking more than RDA's of certain vitamins.

Following are some recent thoughts on the subject. Vitamin A supplements may reduce risk of breast cancer. Vitamin C, extra 300 mg per day, may reduce risk of eye cataracts. Vitamin E, extra 400+ IU per day, may reduce risk of heart disease and may augment cholesterol-lowering medications. On the other hand, some studies show that very large doses of Vitamins A, D, B6 and C seem to cause problems and can interact adversely with prescription medications. For example, doctors advise that foods with Vitamin K (leafy greens) should be avoided by those taking Coumadin for blood clot prevention. This is another topic to discuss with your doctor.

Scientific studies to determine the difference that vitamin supplements make in one's health are very difficult to conduct. This is because there is a problem in having one test group of people with a vitamin supplement and another test group without it, while keeping all other variables (like menu or medication) constant, to determine the difference that the vitamin supplement makes. Because of this difficulty, the value of vitamin supplements is controversial and is likely to remain so for years. In other words, we can't be certain that extra vitamins over the RDA's are beneficial or not. The prevailing view is to take moderate supplements anyway unless it proves to be harmful. There is a belief that excess vitamins are simply passed through the body with no effect. However, as mentioned above, it may be possible to over-dose with some vitamins. The National Academy of Science is conducting studies in that regard. Also, there is growing evidence that vitamin requirements change with age. Better information on this subject should be available in the future. The bottom line for seniors is that vitamins are important for good health. Whether or not they contribute to longevity remains an unanswered question. Incidentally, cases of vitamin deficiency (scurvy, beriberi. pellagra, etc.) which were rather common a century ago are rarely seen in developed countries today.

One matter warrants special comment. Alcohol will destroy or reduce the benefit of most vitamins. Although a glass of wine adds pleasure to the day of many seniors and there is evidence that wine in moderation is beneficial to the heart, any drinking of alcoholic beverages has to be weighed against the loss of value of vitamins. Again, alcoholic beverages contain calories and little or no nutrients. Most soft drinks aren't much better. Unless sugar-free, they are really "candy in a bottle". Water is the dieter's friend. Not only is it calorie-free but it gives the illusion of fullness and reduces the desire for larger or second helpings of food.

Minerals, which are metallic compounds found in soil and water, are also important. Iron compounds, found mostly in certain vegetables like spinach and in some red meats, are essential for creating hemoglobin in the blood. Calcium is needed for strong bones and as a preventative for osteoporosis. The role of other minerals in the diet is not fully known, but they seem to be important. Zinc is believed to be helpful in maintaining good eyesight. The roles of chromium, selenium, magnesium, potassium and copper compounds are uncertain, but some of each is believed to be helpful. There are no RDA's for most minerals. The source of minerals is mainly through grains and vegetables. Since grains and vegetables do not make minerals and they must originate from soil, water or fertilizer and because all soils and water do not provide the needed minerals, eating vegetables grown in a variety of locations is a good idea. Although many producers of flour enrich their product with minerals, this fact does not eliminate the need for taking mineral as well as vitamin supplements.

Before buying a multi-vitamin or mineral supplement, one should discuss the matter with one's physician and ask for his/her recommendation. Vitamin packaging labels carry important information on contents including the % of the Recommended Dietary Allowances (RDA). One should study the label on the package to know the content. It is well known that women are more susceptible than men to osteoporosis and the loss of bone mass due to deficient assimilation of calcium. Calcium supplements are often recommended by doctors. They may also prescribe an ethical drug like Fosamax, Evista or Estrogen to prevent or treat osteoporosis.

The results of further research regarding dietary supplements are being published continually and conventional ideas are sometimes overturned. Seniors should try to stay abreast of these developments. A good way to do this is to read regularly *Prevention Magazine* or the *Nutrition Action Health Letter* which is published monthly by the Center for Science in the Public Interest or medical school newsletters like those from Harvard or Johns Hopkins.

While it is important to know what one should eat, once again, it's also important to know what to avoid. Many fast foods and snack items are loaded with fat and salt. Although some salt and fat is necessary, too much sodium (i.e. salt and some preservatives) is considered harmful. It may be helpful to think of these items as "poisonous".

As an example of the effects of poor eating habits, I often think of my deceased business associate, Len, who used to order two hamburgers and an order of fries every day for lunch. On the fries he'd dump extra salt—always the same. I understand that night after night, it was fried chicken and more fries with beers before and after dinner. After years of this high fat and salt diet, Len developed a big belly and his skin seemed to take on a pale gray tone. Friends tried to warn him, but he liked his favorites and wouldn't change. Len took an early retirement at age 58 and enjoyed 2 years of it before passing on from a heart attack, the result of clogged arteries.

People who would like to weigh less probably have to think differently about food. Those who grew up in the Depression years may recall the adage, "he who wastes shall want". One needs to think instead, "Better in the waste than on the waist". Although being overweight is the concern of many seniors, there are some who have the opposite problem—being underweight and frail. Perhaps they need to eat more of high-calorie foods. However, anyone who is either overweight or underweight should discuss the matter with their doctor before adopting a different diet. They might have a more serious problem than weight.

Thoughts on Exercise and Physical Activity

In view of all the publicity, there can be hardly anyone who doesn't already realize that exercise is important for good health and physical condition. For those who wish to go into their elder years able to enjoy life and to have physical options, doing something physical every day is like having money in the bank. As the old saying goes, "If you don't use it, you lose it".

If exercise is so important, why doesn't everyone do it? The answers might range from: it takes too much time, it makes me tired, I don't like the feeling of sweating and straining, it's boring, or I'd rather sleep, read, eat or watch TV. Couch potatoes come in all sizes and ages. It's not a state reserved for the beat generation. Sofa spuds may not live as long or maintain wellness. Worst of all, little in the way of self satisfaction is likely to come to those who spend much of their day slumped in a recliner watching TV and gobbling junk food.

Many of those who exercise faithfully don't always enjoy it. They do it because they know that it's good for their general health and the physical options like adventure travel and independence that it brings. Exercise doesn't mean marathon running or even lots of tennis. There are milder forms of beneficial exercise. In fact, running and tennis may be rather hard on aging joints.

For those who are able, probably the best all-around conditioning exercises are swimming, bicycling, brisk walking or cross-country skiing. All enable the participant to get the heart beating at an elevated level for an extended period of time. For general conditioning, a typical senior should get his/her pulse up to between 100 and 120 beats per minute for at least 15 minutes, 3 times per week. Swimming and bicycling are good in that the body weight is supported and there is little pressure on the joints. Walking that is brisk enough to raise the pulse is both convenient (often right out the front door) and interesting (as one observes the neighborhood or other scenery). Mall walking is also interesting and is a great refuge in unpleasant weather. Uphill walking truly raises the spirit as well as body and pulse. An alternative is going up and down your household stairway. These are steps not worth saving. In fact, it has been said that each step up adds 4 seconds to one's life span. Cross-country skiing is probably the best of all exercises because it works multiple parts of the body and is non-jarring on knees and hips. However, in most parts of the country and most seasons of the year, one will have to settle for a stationary ski machine. Stationary bikes and treadmills are good alternatives.

The biggest problem is the self-discipline required to exercise faithfully. As in dieting, one can call upon one's spiritual resources to help. You might keep telling yourself that exercise is good for the soul as well as the body.

Joining a health club or community seniors' exercise class may help to inspire regularity. Also, most gym facilities have a variety of equipment designed to strengthen the major muscle groups while alleviating boredom. Most clubs offer aerobic classes with maneuvers that are done to music. That plus the sociability can make it all a pleasant experience. Also most health clubs have trainers available who can custom-design an exercise program. Alternatively, exercise machines like stationary bikes, treadmills or ski machines purchased for use at home make exercise convenient and monotony can be eased by TV watching or reading while doing your good deed for yourself for the day.

There are many excellent exercises that involve a minimum of equipment. Cans of soup can serve as bar bells for arm and shoulder workouts. Old panty hose or a heavy elastic can be stretch resistance for leg and back exercises. Just plain body weight is often resistance enough for squats or sit-ups.

There are more than 50 books currently in print on the subject of fitness for seniors. Below is a sample of the exercises they suggest. As with dieting, your doctor should be consulted before starting an exercise program because an inappropriate selection can cause back pain or heart strain.

1. Warm up with an arm stretch reaching over your ear down behind your back one arm at a time as far as you can. Hold it for a few seconds. Repeat 10 times

2. Lie flat on the floor and pull one knee at a time up to your chest and hold for a few seconds. Repeat 10 times.

3. Throw 10 coins on the floor and bend over and pick them up one by one while keeping legs as straight as possible and standing upright in between picks.

4. Loop a panty hose or exercise elastic around a bedpost at chest height. With arms straight, pull backward to flex back muscles and hold for a few seconds. Repeat 10 times. This may help to improve one's posture.

5. Hold a full soup can in each hand and raise sideways to above your shoulder and hold for a few seconds. Repeat 10 times.

6. With a soup can in each hand, arms straight ahead, curl arms upward to shoulders. Repeat until tired.

7. With hose or elastic around ankles, spread feet outward. Lie back and press outward. Repeat until tired.

8. Facing away from wall and about a foot away, twist upper body around and touch wall with both hands. First one side then the other. Repeat 10 times.

Just these few exercises done every day will help to retain one's flexibility and avoid some aches due to muscular fatigue.

You may check in your local library or bookstore for books with detailed descriptions of a variety of exercises, many of which are designed to strengthen certain muscle groups. Backaches may be prevented by having a healthy back as the result of faithful exercises to strengthen and flex it. In cases of back pain, one might consult a chiropractor for treatment and analysis. Your family doctor may also prescribe muscle-relaxants to relieve back pain or, for persistent problems, he/she may find that back surgery is required to relieve the pain. A podiatrist may detect that foot problems are causing an imbalance that leads to back pain.

Housework can be good exercise for those who are able and willing. Bending and reaching or shoving a vacuum cleaner back and forth can be aerobically beneficial. Going up and down stairs is an excellent conditioner. If stair climbing is necessary by virtue of where you live or how your home is designed, you can appreciate the exercise value. You could make extra trips just for the fun of it.

If you are physically disabled or if exercises like those above are inappropriate, you can do isometric exercises. Isometrics are muscle flexings or pressure exertion with no motion.

Isometrics can be done while sitting in a chair, standing in line, waiting in an airport or riding on a bus or plane. Here are a few examples:

1. Push against the palms of your hands with each other as hard as you can. Hold until it begins to hurt.

2. Do the same only pull with curled fingers.

3. While sitting, push on the floor as hard as you can with both legs without raising the body. Hold until it starts to hurt.

4. Grasping the arms of your chair, push hard enough to raise your body a little. Hold until it starts to hurt.

While exercise is very good for improving strength, condition and balance, it's not the easiest way to lose weight. It takes an enormous amount of exercise (like walking more than 25 miles on the level) to lose a pound of fat. The best weight-losing exercise is to push yourself away from the table or walk past the dessert tray looking straight ahead. However, exercise and/or being physically active combined with diet helps to convert fat to muscle. Exercise also tends to convert LDL (bad cholesterol) to HDL (good cholesterol).

For both dieting and exercise, some kind of inspiration is needed to keep doing what is difficult or somewhat unpleasant. Think of the discomfort as a "character builder". You'll feel better and proud of yourself and others will admire you. Isn't that sufficient reward?

Sexual Fulfillment for Seniors

Some of us with a 1930's mentality may be uncomfortable discussing this subject even though sexuality is a very basic human characteristic and a topic that still interests many seniors. The question, "Is there sex after sixty?" is often asked. According to Dr. Ruth Westheimer, men and women can experience orgasms up to age 100. Is that useful information? While some may say "hooray", others may feel guilt or remorse or maybe even disgust because they can't abide or don't feel like participating. This is a personal choice that needs no justification. Dr. Dean Edell, the radio talk show host, claims that sex after sixty is better than ever for many because of lack of fear of pregnancy, less anxiety, more "know how" and enough time to relax and avoid a rush to work or other duties.

Is sex all that important for seniors? Did anyone ever die from lack of sex? No, but, according to Dr. Susan Landolphi, consultant for the Third Age Media, orgasms are good for the immune system, the heart, insomnia and sinus congestion in addition to providing psychic renewal. Whether couples or singles, Dr. Landolphi says that men and women should learn all the ways to generate orgasms for themselves and each other. For more information, read her book, *The Best Love, the Best Sex: Creating Sensual, Soulful, Supersatisfying Relationships.*

Also, Virginia Johnson Masters of the Masters & Johnson Institute for sexuality research states that sex improves skin tone and color. She claims that the risk of prostate cancer is reduced for men who ejaculate on a regular basis. She adds that sex stimulates endorphin release, which enables one to sleep more soundly and gives one a general feeling of well-being. Moreover, sex is a good cardiovascular workout. She also says that one should never presume that sex is only physical; it is a mind/body/spirit experience. Dr. M. Scott Peck, author of the best-seller, *Further Along the Road Less Traveled*, adds that orgasms are mystic and spiritual and the ultimate mind-body interaction.

More than one senior has said, "Sex simply isn't worth the trouble any more". For seniors who may find customary sexual activity too taxing, uncomfortable or painful, Dr. Landolphi suggests alternative ways to relieve the "trouble". She says that many senior couples seem to be oblivious to the idea that sexual intimacy can keep long marriages from becoming tired and dull. She goes on to point out that satisfying sexual intimacy can mean just close holding and touching without intercourse. Regarding the exertion concern, weight control and exercise, in addition to being good for one's general physical condition and health, should help extend an active sex life. Fitness may have a bearing on one's libido as well. What more can be said about Viagra that hasn't already been overdone.

Dr. Ruth Westheimer, along with many other experts, says that when both members of a relationship keep their libido, are in good shape physically and mentally, the sparks can fly for years. However, if both members of a couple have lost their libido and a disinterest in sex is mutual, they probably do not view themselves as unfortunate. Problems can arise, however, when one member of a couple has a libido that is still strong while the other's has lapsed. For this problem there are no easy solutions and seeing a family therapist is advised. Widow(er)s and other older singles may still have a strong libido that may require some creativity to remedy. Answers to these concerns may also be found in Dr. Landolphi's book. Dr. Edell also points out that the brain is the paramount sex organ. He says that seniors with disabilities that make customary sex acts difficult, painful or unpleasant should learn that intimate and creative touching and stroking together with whispered suggestions can be effective in adding excitement to a life that is in danger of becoming dull.

Writing in *Psychology Today*, Shirley Glass indicates that infidelity among long-married seniors is more common than might be expected. It comes about when one member of a couple has mental or physical deterioration and the other wishes for wholeness in his/her life. Finding emotional nurturing with another person can happen with no loss of commitment to the spouse and it may be an emotional, not physical, relationship with the other person.

Dr. C. Marrett Lacey suggests that a good marriage or relationship must have intimacy and friendship as well as commitment and that when any part of the mix is lost due to age-related weariness or loss of faculties, an urge to regain emotional nurturing is a natural result.

In summary, important factors for a fulfilling Third Age are weight control, good nutrition, proper mental and physical medical care, exercise and a satisfying sex life. These things don't "just happen". They must be addressed with planning, initiative and determination. A quest for spiritual growth can be the inspiration for the determination and enhanced spirituality can be the reward for success.

"To age well is not an accident.
It is a gift that those who care can give to themselves."

—Stephen T. Gullo, PhD

VI

END OF LIFE DECISIONS

Exit Gracefully by: Planning a Funeral and Disposition of Remains; Making Wills and Bequests; Writing an Obituary; Executing Living Wills, Health-Care Proxies and Empowerment Letters. For survivors—Dealing with Grief and Finding a New Life.

Although never a pleasant topic, the end of life is an inevitability to face and plan for. I think it would be nice if, when my time is up, I could simply take a bow to the audience, step behind a curtain amid their applause and vanish. Unfortunately it doesn't work that way. Writer Pamela Sebastian describes "good" deaths and "bad" deaths. The good death comes to those who view the end with courage, acceptance and a willingness to talk about it; a bad death is accompanied by denial, dread and a desperate attempt to hang on. Probably more than any other time in life, faith in what comes next is needed at this hour. As the line from the hymn "Amazing Grace" says, "Faith will see us through".

Planning a Funeral and Disposition of Remains

The Christian Creed ends with "I believe in the resurrection of the body and life everlasting. Amen." For those that hold a literal view of "resurrection of the body", burial of the whole body is probably the chosen method of disposition of remains in order to facilitate the rising from the dead. Those who believe that "resurrection of the body" is a metaphor think that a human cannot be reconstituted to life as we know it. Instead, they believe that it's the spirit that has eternal life and they regard cremation or some other form of treating bodily remains acceptable, although they might still prefer bodily burial. Upon death, some people would like to offer their organs for transplants or their bodies for medical research or education. Others may chose cremation as a way to save burial space and expense. This is a personal choice that should be communicated, in writing, to survivors or next of kin who have the responsibility for final arrangements.

As a resting-place for remains, there is the conventional cemetery plot, a vault or a scattering of ashes over some special place. Cemetery land is becoming difficult to acquire in many localities and vaults or columbaria are becoming a preferred option. A plot with a monument provides a place for friends and relatives to contemplate a lost loved-one or for descendants to learn about forebears many years hence. If one's choice is a cemetery burial, it is advisable to contract for the plot long before one thinks they will need it. Predetermined arrangements spare the family of hasty, emotional decisions at an inopportune time.

A funeral is for the benefit of those left behind and they have the last word regarding the event. Those anticipating death may wish to describe the service, music, readings and participation or even an after-funeral gathering. These choices should be put in writing and made available to those who will take care of the arrangements. Others may have lived in denial to the end and expressed no disposal wishes whatsoever. Those left behind may wish to honor the departed with a major procession. Still others may prefer to have the affair as inconspicuous as possible. Still other next of kin may abandon the departed altogether. More than one relative has left a funeral director without instructions regarding disposition of the remains and they lie unclaimed with the funeral director. A San Diego firm offers to blast remains into the heavens out of a cannon with optional fireworks. What next?

Wills and Bequests

Is there any senior who doesn't realize that he/she should have a will if they have any property at all to leave behind? Most seniors give their wills a high priority and perhaps years of thought, yet many die each year intestate, leaving disposition of assets to the decision of the Probate Court. A will should be carefully drawn, most likely by a lawyer with all contingencies covered. It should be current, duly executed and witnessed. It is not the intent here to define how to make a will except to say that it should be done while one is of sound mind. It should be written unambiguously so that it will not be contested by heirs or beneficiaries and should take into account the intention and wishes of the departed. Perhaps the reason that some seniors have not made wills or kept them current is that they don't care what becomes of their assets. Maybe there are few assets; maybe no close heirs; maybe the logical heirs are perceived as contrary, rude, selfish or have an objectionable life style. Wills are a way to make a statement. Some autocrats may even try to "rule from the grave" through their wills.

Lawyers are not perfect. There are instances when a will has been composed by a lawyer in a hurry and who has not provided for all contingencies or has inadvertently induced contradictions. This is especially cogent if there is a trust that will be distributed many years in the future when many situations may have changed. Also, a good lawyer is also an estate planner and will have had his/her client arrange financial matters well before one's death to minimize estate taxes, if any. If there is a lot at stake or there are family complications, a second legal opinion and/or that of a tax expert may be useful. Also, state laws vary and, if one might die in a different state, it may be necessary to have a second lawyer in the other state.

A will is an opportunity to thank and care for faithful and loving friends and relatives and to endow favorite charities. The first priority is usually a surviving spouse, then the children. A reason for deviating from that pattern may be that the spouse does not need more money and a bequest to the spouse would mainly add to the spouse's taxable estate. This is especially true if the spouse's longevity expectation is relatively short. If the children are well-off financially, it may make sense to skip them and leave money to the grandchildren instead. Perhaps one child needs the money more than another or was a sacrificing caregiver. These are a couple of reasons for treating children unequally. It might be a good idea to explain such an inequality in the will to reduce the likelihood of hurt feelings. The possibilities of complex issues like these are myriad. A good lawyer will help one through the logic to arrive at a fair arrangement.

In may make sense for a person who has significant wealth to make major bequests while alive rather than by will. Not only might taxes be reduced, but also one can enjoy appreciation and see the fruits of their lifetime of effort. On the other hand, most people would rather not give away so much that they outlive their resources and become dependent on others. Again, if you knew exactly how long you'd live and had a good idea of all your expenses in the meantime, you could arrange to spend your last dollar the day you die. Lacking that knowledge, one should keep adequate reserves to the end. Although it may sound surreptitious, seniors in failing health may hold out the promise of a bequest as an incentive for caregivers. Toward the end, one's money may be the only power one has left. This is, perhaps, another reason for not spending the last dollar of one's resources.

Writing an Obituary

Among the practical things that you might want to do while lucid is to compose an obituary for yourself and have it available when needed. It should include those activities and works for which you'd like to be remembered expressed in the way you want. Don't expect a grieving spouse to take on this chore at a most inopportune time. Similarly, don't expect your children to do it the way you'd like. They might not even get the facts correct. Make it as lengthy as you think the local paper will print. The funeral director should arrange for the publication. Also, the content might be useful to a survivor or minister in preparing a eulogy.

Living Wills, Health Care Proxies and Empowerment Letters

Although many seniors are realistic enough not to fear death, they might worry about the dying process. Dying can be painful, expensive and a burden to caregivers. Fortunate are those like my Uncle Jack who, at age 93, went swimming at Fire Island, came home and expired while sitting by the fire, happy in the midst of his family. Most people aren't that fortunate.

On average, something like one half of one's lifetime medical expenses are incurred in the last year of one's life. Big medical expenses usually correlate with considerable pain and discomfort. Some people will agonize over the expense with the thought that the money could be better used in other ways, for example, to help pay for a grandchild's education. A clear view on this subject is held by the Hemlock Society that believes that when a person has a painful terminal illness with no hope of recovery, euthanasia is a practical alternative. Of course this idea is subject to much controversy, many will disdain the notion altogether and some states prohibit the practice. For more information on this subject, one should contact the Hemlock Society at Box 101810, Denver, CO 80250. There are about 25 other organizations in the country that advocate the "death with dignity" concept.

A more moderate approach to end-of-life decisions is the Living Will. These written instruments are fairly standard and some prototypes have a checklist of optional life-sustaining measures that can be refused in the event of a terminal and painful illness. They might say that there should be no artificial resuscitation, no heart-lung machine, no antibiotics, no intravenous or forced feeding or hydration. If one feels this way, a signed document should be prepared and be in the files of your primary care physician, attending doctor and lawyer with copies to anyone else who might be concerned. Again, this Will should be composed and witnessed while one is of a sound mind.

A supplement to the Living Will is the Health-Care Proxy. This is a document that authorizes another person to decide whether or not life support is to be provided to the named person who is terminally ill and has lost the ability to communicate. It may be better to give this power to a trusted and willing friend who understands your wishes and may be less likely to be swayed by emotion than a member of your family.

These documents, nevertheless, may not be honored by some hospitals or nursing homes for fear that there may be some relative who might object and would sue the doctor and/or the institution. As mentioned earlier, for this contingency, Dr. Timothy Quill urges will-makers to compose a letter of empowerment that gives to a family member or heir the right to bring suit against any hospital or nursing home that does not abide by one's Living Will or Proxy. All of these documents should be updated about every 7 years.

Dealing With Grief and Finding a New Life

The death of a spouse or partner is often one of the most traumatic experiences of a lifetime even if it is expected. Some cope well; others do not. There is little that can be said to dispel the sadness of a grieving survivor at that time, however prayer is often comforting to strong believers. In any event, it is a good idea to have a "support system" in place. This may be a network of family and friends or a church. It's doubly difficult if one has to deal with grief by oneself.

Recovery from the death of a loved-one has to be mostly self-generated. An unexpected death may be worse than one that has been anticipated. If one has watched their spouse/partner decline in health over a period of time, there has been an opportunity to plan for the eventuality and think about what comes next. Even then, denial or false hope can get in the way of the inevitable adjustment. It is better to face the future realistically and be prepared.

A death that occurs unexpectedly is especially upsetting when the surviving partner has been highly dependent on the departed partner for many aspects of practical living. In that case, the sadness of losing a lover, friend, partner and confidant is compounded by the loss of capacity to deal with life's realities. One not only has to work through the grief but must also learn to handle the host of duties that the departed spouse/partner may have managed.

Obviously, this problem has been faced by countless millions before us. Some cope well; a few feel suicidal; most muddle through. Fortunate are those who have compassionate clergy, friends or children that are helpful at this critical time. Fewer and fewer of us have helpful children who live nearby. Many must deal with grief plus adjustment alone.

One way to think about the situation is to view the death of a spouse/partner as a transition—hopefully, a transition to a satisfying new life. Here are some typical, sequential steps that can be followed after the death to reduce the anxiety of the transition:

1. Notify your family doctor, minister, family members and close friends and a (previously selected) funeral director. If possible, recruit friends and family to help with this.

2. Work with the funeral director to make funeral arrangements including tasks like casket or urn selection. Work with clergy person to plan ceremony.

3. Attend the service and try to make attendees comfortable.

4. Notify your lawyer, insurance agents, banks, Social Security and any former employer from whom benefits are being received. If you are not the executor of the estate, notify the person named as executor in the will.

5. Take time out for grieving. Maybe take a trip or spend time with close friends and family. If it is your practice, say prayers of thanksgiving for the life of the deceased person and for strength to deal with your own future.

6. Make a list of all the duties that the spouse took care of. Often what comes in the mail is a reminder of taxes due and bills to be paid. Especially, have a handle on tax payments and other regular bills for which late payment bears a penalty. Have a list of all household maintenance requirements.

7. Be sure to eat nutritiously and on time. Avoid drinking alcohol alone—it may make matters worse.

8. Dispose of the deceased person's clothing and personal items. This may be the most wrenching action for a survivor. Try to get help from family or close friends with this. They may be comforting as well as helpful.

9. Think about alternative places to live, especially if there are difficult financial or maintenance considerations in the present location. However, take lots of time, maybe a year or more, to study options. Don't hastily move in with children unless necessary for

financial reasons; they have problems of their own. If moving is the sensible thing to do, study alternatives before making a decision, then plan the move.

10.If moving is appropriate, dispose of unneeded belongings through sale or gifts; select the new dwelling; put present dwelling (if there is one) up for sale; make the move and settle in.

11.Look over the list of activities in Chapter III of this book for ideas and plan a new life going forward.

12.Be proactive in finding new friends to fill the void of the lost spouse/partner.

13.After the grieving has subsided and when ready, be open to developing a relationship with one of the opposite sex. (This is not a betrayal of the lost spouse. One can loyally love two people.)

14.Consider remarriage, but perhaps a partnership or companionship would be better. Re-read the section on friendship and prenuptial agreements in Chapter IV.

After-death adjustments are difficult, to be sure, but a spiritually-inspired outlook can lead to a satisfying and fulfilling outcome.

Conclusion

To restate things, the purpose of this book is to take a look at the major issues that persons over 60 are likely to face. A Third Age, lasting 30 years or so, lies ahead for many and they will encounter a number of these issues. This book has tried to say something relevant and helpful about these issues and encourage Third Agers to make the most of this time so it will be fulfilling, interesting, enjoyable and spiritually uplifting. The Third Age is a time to harvest what we have been growing and tending all these years. It can be the most meaningful time of life. A strong emphasis on spirituality has been woven into this book. The concept is offered that the "next life" is one of the spirit. For those who are comfortable with this idea, it is suggested that the more a person has grown spiritually in their Third Age, the more glorious will be their spirit among the departed.

The content of this book could be called an anthology or a condensation of the range of senior issues. Much supplementary reading about and/or group discussion of the various issues is suggested. Personal experiences regarding all these issues shared with both old friends and new acquaintances can be supportive and enlightening. It is hoped that the ideas expressed in this book will make a difference in the personal life of the reader.

"All's well that ends well"

—Wm. Shakespeare

READING LIST

Mind/Spirit/Wellness Interaction

Timeless Healing: The Power and Biology of Belief
Herbert Benson, M.D. 1996

Healing Words: Prayer is Good Medicine
Larry Dossey, M.D. 1995

Science and Health, with Key to the Scriptures
Mary Baker Eddy 1875 (1997)

The Measure of Our Days: A Spiritual Exploration of Wellness
Jerome Groopman 1998

Stopping the Clock
Dr. Ronald Klatz and Dr. Robert Goldman 1996

Religion in Aging and Health: Theological Foundations and Methodological Frontiers
J.S. Levin 1994

The Longevity Strategy: How to Live to 100 Using the Brain-Body Connection
David Mahoney and Richard Restak, M.D. 1998

The Faith Factor: Proof of the Healing Power of Prayer
Dale A. Matthews, M.D. 1993

The Nine Myths of Aging: Maximizing the Quality of Later Life
Douglas H. Powell 1998

Love, Medicine & Miracles: Lessons Learned About Self-Healing from a Surgeon's Experience with Exceptional Patients
Bernie Siegel, M.D. 1990

Spirituality

Mid-Life-Psychological and Spiritual Perspectives
Janice Brewi and Anne Brenneab 1997

The Seven Spiritual Laws of Success
Deepak Chopra 1997

The Road Less Traveled—A New Psychology of Love, Traditional Values and Spiritual Growth
M. Scott Peck, M.D. 1978

Further Along the Road Less Traveled—The Unending Journey Toward Spiritual Growth
M. Scott Peck, M.D. 1993

Personal Finance

Graham & Dodd's Security Analysis
Sidney Cottle, Frank E. Block and Roger F. Murray 1988

One Up on Wall Street
Peter Lynch 1991

Beating the Street
Peter Lynch 1994

The Wall Street Journal Guide to Understanding Money and Investing
Kenneth M. Morris and Alan M. Siegel 1994

Nine Steps to Financial Freedom
Suze Orman 1997

You've Earned It Don't Lose It: Mistakes You Can't Afford to Make When You Retire
Suze Orman & Linda Mead 1997

The Courage to be Rich: Creating a Life of Material and Spiritual Abundance
Suze Orman 1999

Diet & Exercise

Arthritis of the Hip & Knee—An Active Person's Guide to Taking Charge

Ronald J. Allen, Victoria Anne Brander, M.D. and S. David Stuberg, M.D. 1998

Eat Right for Your Type: The Individualized Diet Solution to Staying Healthy Living Longer and Achieving Your Ideal Weight
Peter J. D'Amando, M.D. 1996

The Complete Book of Fitness: Mind, Body, Spirit
Karen Andes 1995

An Eating Plan for Healthy Americans
American Heart Association

The American Dietetic Association's Complete Food & Nutrition Guide
Roberta Larson Duyff 1996

It's Never Too Late to Look and Feel Younger Through Exercise
Oliver Heuts 1997

Strong Women Stay Young
Miriam E. Nelson, Ph.D. 1997

Death and Dying

The Measure of Our Days: New Beginnings at Life's End
Jerome Groodman 1997

On Death and Dying
Elizabeth Kubler-Ross, M.D. 1997

How We Die: Reflecting on Life's Final Chapter
Sherwin B. Nuland 1995

Aging and Eldering

Dare to be 100
Walter M. Bortz 1996

Virtues of Aging
Jimmy Carter 1998

Ageless Body. Timeless Mind
Deepak Chopra 1993

Successful Aging
Jack Rome, M.D. and Robert L. Kahn 1998

From Aqe-ing to Sage-ing: A Profound New Vision of Growing Older
Zalman Schacter-Shalomi and Ron Miller 1997

Sexuality

Love and Sex after 60
Robert Butler, MD and Myrna Lewis 1993

*The Best Love, the Best Sex: Creating Sensual, Soulful
Supersatisfying-Relationships*
Susan Landolphi, Ph.D. 1997

The Soul of Sex: Cultivating Life as an Act of Love
Thomas Moore 1998

*I'm Not in the Mood–What Every Woman Should Know About Improving Her
Libido*
Judith Reichman, M.D. 1998

Other Topics of Interest to Seniors

Secrets of Becoming a Late Bloomer
Connie Goldmon and Richard Mahler 1995

The Last Gift of Time: Life Beyond 60
Carolyn Heilbrun 1997

Grandparenting Long Distance: 35 Ways to Keep in Touch & Keep Love Alive
Gwenyth Kerr 1996

The Book of Myself: A Do-It-Yourslf Autobiography in 201 Questions
Carl Marshall and David Marshall 1997

Remembering Your Story: A Guide to Spiritual Autobiography
Richard L. Morgan 1996

Take Care of Yourself–The Complete Illustrated Guide to Medical Self-Care 6th
Edition
Donald M. Vickery, M.D. and James F. Fries, M.D. 1997

Granparenthood
Ruth Westheimer, M.D. and Steven Kaplan 1998

About the Author

William N. (Bill) Hosley was born in Newton, Massachusetts in 1925. He attended Dartmouth College and the University of Rochester and was graduated from the Sloan School of Industrial Management at the Massachusetts Institute of Technology in 1948. He served in the Naval Air Corps during WWII. He has lived with his wife in Rochester, NY since 1948 and is the father of three adult sons and has two grandchildren.

His business career, which has not yet ended, has included professional and management experience in human relations, finance, marketing and industrial research. He is the author of four books on subjects as diverse as winemaking, economics, project management and local history. He has been an adjunct university professor and guest lecturer on business subjects. In addition, he has published many articles on mental health, mathematics, quality improvement and computer applications. He is an investment advisor registered by the Securities & Exchange Commission. Currently, he is on the boards of three mental health service providers and a member of their quality improvement and human values committees. He has traveled extensively and is an enthusiastic skier, mountain climber, tennis player and boater. He has been active in church affairs for many years and is currently a member of the adult education committees of several community organizations in Rochester.

He continues to enjoy adventures and still has a number of dreams to follow. Moreover, he likes the feeling that he has more control over his life in his Third Age than ever before. He wishes the same for all seniors.

9 781583 482896